T0257419

# Practical Transfusion Medicine

## for the Small Animal Practitioner

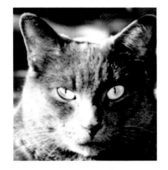

Bernard F. Feldman
DVM, Ph.D. (Deceased)
Formerly, Chief, Laboratory Diagnostic Services
Virginia-Maryland Regional College of Veterinary Medicine
Blacksburg, Maryland

Carolyn A. Sink
MS, MT (ASCP)
Supervisor, Laboratory Diagnostic Services
Virginia-Maryland Regional College of Veterinary Medicine
Blacksburg, Maryland

Photographs by:
Donna L. Burton CLS (NCA)

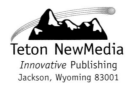

Teton NewMedia
*Innovative* Publishing
Jackson, Wyoming 83001

Executive Editor: Carroll C. Cann
Development Editor: Susan L. Hunsberger
Creative Director: Sue Haun 5640 Design, www.fiftysixforty.com
Production & Layout: Mike Albiniak 5640 Design, www.fiftysixforty.com
Photographs: Donna L. Burton CLS (NCA)


Teton NewMedia
P.O. Box 4833
90 East Simpson Street
Jackson, WY 83001
1-888-770-3165
www.tetonnewmedia.com

PRINTED IN THE UNITED STATES OF AMERICA

ISBN 1-893441-04-0

Print number 5 4 3 2 1

    Library of Congress Cataloging–in–Publication Data

Feldman, Bernard F. (Bernard Frank)
    Practical transfusion medicine for small animal practitioners / Bernard F. Feldman,
Carolyn Sink.
       p, ; cm. —(Made easy series)
    Includes Index.
    ISBN 1–893441–04–0 (alk paper)
    1. Dogs--Diseases--Treatment. 2. Cats--Disease--Treatment. 3. Veterinary hematology
4. Blood--Transfusion. I. Sink, Carloyn A. II. Title. III. Made easy series (Jackson Wyo.)
    [DNLM: 1. Blood Banks--organization & administration. 2. Blood
Transfusion--veterinary. 3. Animals, Domestic. 4. Blood Specimen Collection--veterinary.]
SF992.B57F45 2004
636.089'615--dc22

                                                                2004062050

# Dedication

This book is dedicated to the memory of Dr. Bernard F. Feldman.

Carolyn Sink
Donna Burton

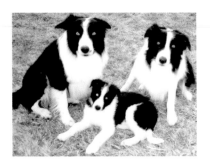

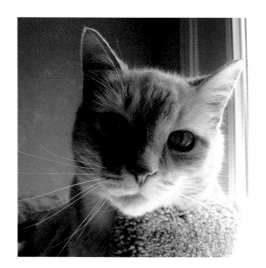

# Acknowledgment

Recognizing that no technical book is completely the original work of the authors, I would like to express my appreciation to everyone who gave me direction and helped me understand what would be most clinically useful on a day to day basis.

Special thanks to Donna Burton and Dr. William Swecker, Jr.

Carolyn Sink

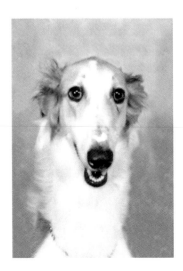

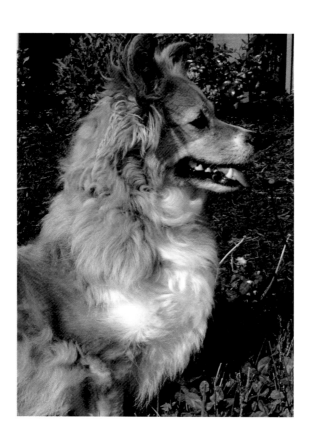

# Preface

Interest in transfusion medicine by veterinary professionals was first recorded at the 87th Annual Meeting of the American Veterinary Medical Association in 1950. Since this time, advances in human transfusion medicine have led to advances in veterinary transfusion medicine. One benefit of this technology has been in blood component therapy. Separation of a unit of whole blood into components was made possible by the development of plastic bags for blood collection and high speed refrigerated centrifuges. Manipulation of whole into blood components is a relatively simple task and this text has been created to highlight the fundamental principles of blood bank techniques. We have included fuller procedures of some critical requirements for accuracy and service to the needs of our patients.

Bernard Feldman
Carolyn Sink

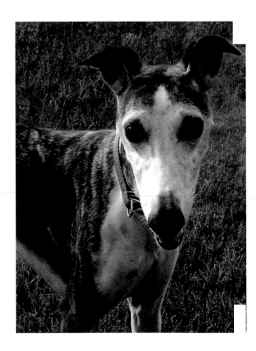

# Table of Contents

## Section 1 Creation of a Community Based Blood Bank

Introduction. . . . . . . . . . . . . . . . . . . . . . . 3
Some Helpful Hints. . . . . . . . . . . . . . . . . 3
Owner Recruitment. . . . . . . . . . . . . . . . . 4
Owner and Donor Attributes . . . . . . . . . . 5
Basic Equipment Needs for Blood
Collection, Processing and Storage. . . . . . . . . . 10

## Section 2 Blood Collection Systems, Processing, Storage and Shipment

Anticoagulants and Preservatives . . . . . . . . . . . 16
Blood Collection Systems . . . . . . . . . . . . . . . 18
Blood Product Overview . . . . . . . . . . . . . . . 21
Blood Collection Systems and
Pre-Processing Guidelines . . . . . . . . . . . . . 26
Preparation of Fresh Whole Blood . . . . . . . . . 29
Preparation of Red Cells and
Fresh Frozen Plasma. . . . . . . . . . . . . . . . 29
Preparation of Cryoprecipitated
Anti-Hemophilic Factor and
Cryo-Poor Plasma . . . . . . . . . . . . . . . . . 35
Preparation of Platelet Rich Plasma . . . . . . . . . 37
Short Draw and Decreasing the
Amount of Anticoagulant Preservative . . . . . . . . 39
Purchasing and Receiving Blood Products
from Outside Sources. . . . . . . . . . . . . . . . 40
Preparing Blood Products for Shipment . . . . . . . 42

# Section 3 Clinical Considerations in Transfusion Practice

The Crossmatch. . . . . . . . . . . . . . . . . . . . . 46
Blood Transfusion Guidelines . . . . . . . . . . . . . . 47
Blood Substitutes: Alternatives to
Blood and Blood Products. . . . . . . . . . . . . . . . 51
Compatible IV Solutions. . . . . . . . . . . . . . . . . 53
Blood Administration Sets . . . . . . . . . . . . . . . 54
Adverse Effects of Blood Transfusion . . . . . . . . . 55

# Section 4 Biosafety

Laboratory Safety. . . . . . . . . . . . . . . . . . . . 64
Quality Assurance . . . . . . . . . . . . . . . . . . . 65
Records. . . . . . . . . . . . . . . . . . . . . . . . . 67
Inventory Management . . . . . . . . . . . . . . . . . 69

# Section 5 Methods

Preparation of Fresh Whole Blood . . . . . . . . . . . 74
Preparation of Red Cells and
Fresh Frozen Plasma. . . . . . . . . . . . . . . . . . 75
Preparation of Cryoprecipitate and
Cryoprecipitate-Poor Plasma. . . . . . . . . . . . . . 79
Preparation of Platelet Rich Plasma . . . . . . . . . . 80
Crossmatch Procedure . . . . . . . . . . . . . . . . . 83
Washed Cell Suspension . . . . . . . . . . . . . . . . 87
Reaction Grading. . . . . . . . . . . . . . . . . . . . 88
Saline Replacement Procedure . . . . . . . . . . . . . 91
Warming Whole Blood, Red Cells or
Thawing FFP, Cryo or Cryo-Poor Plasma . . . . . . . 93
Centrifuge Calibration. . . . . . . . . . . . . . . . . 95

Appendix 1 Manufacturers
of Blood Collection Bags . . . . . . . . . . . 99

Appendix 2 Organizations
with Veterinary Blood Bank
Interests . . . . . . . . . . . . . . . . . . . . . . . . . . . . . 100

Index . . . . . . . . . . . . . . . . . . . . . . . . . . . . . . . 101

Recommended Readings . . . . . . . . . . . 111

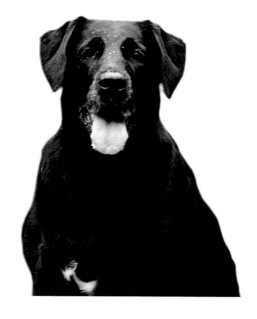

# Section 1

# Creation of a Community Based Blood Bank

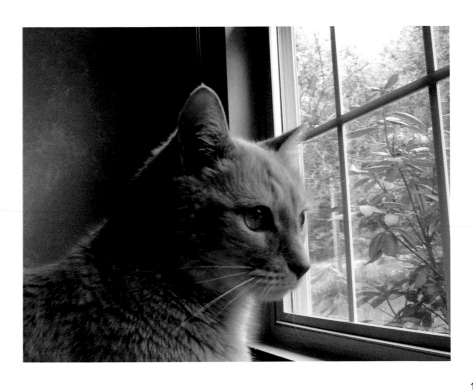

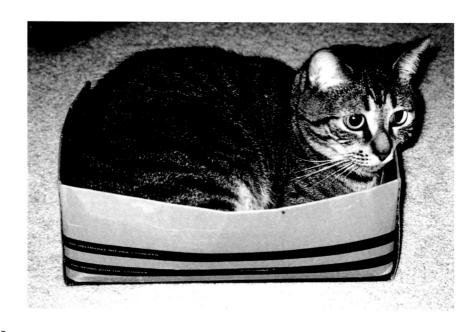

# Introduction

The main goal of this book is to provide an easily readable and accessible reference text which we hope will be readily found on the laboratory bench and will be constantly open and used.

# Some Helpful Hints

Scattered throughout this text are the following symbols to help you focus on what is really important.

✓ This is a routine feature of the subject being discussed. We've tried to narrow them down.

♥ This is an important feature. You should remember this.

💣 Something serious will happen if you do not remember this.

# Owner Recruitment

✔ Owners can be recruited to enlist their pet(s) in to a blood donor program in a variety of ways. This includes:

- Posting notices in the lobby of veterinary clinics
- Advertising in the newspaper
- Advertising at local fairs
- Posting notices at the local human blood center
- By mentioning the need for blood donors to clients
- Advertising to kennel clubs
- Recruiting police dogs

✔ It may be necessary to provide incentives to owners for having their pet(s) in the blood donor program. This may include:

- Discount or free vaccines
- Discount or free flea preventative
- Discount or free heartworm preventative
- Monetary credit for incurred hospital fees
- Discount or free bag of pet food per blood donation
- Free t-shirts for the owners, pet leashes or collars with the practice's logo may provide for advertisement as well as incentive for the program.

✔ Photographs of the blood donors may be posted in the lobby of the veterinary clinic to provide for advertisement to prospective owners as well as recognition of blood donors currently enrolled in the program.

✔ Good communication between owner and practice is critical to the success of the blood donor program. It is very important to specify to the owner exactly what is expected from the owner and donor.

✔ This information may be provided to the owner by creating a written agreement or a "Frequently Asked Questions" brochure. Some items to be included are:

- Routine blood collection dates and times
- The total volume of the blood donation
- The frequency of the blood donation
- How many times per year the blood donor is expected to donate blood
- If the donor is expected to be available for emergency blood donations
- The owner should be informed that a small area on the donor's neck will be shaved and used as the venipuncture site.

✓ It is advisable to specify what fees will be paid by the blood collection facility, and what fees will be billed to the client, including provisions for investigation of abnormal physical examination findings or complications from phlebotomy.

# Owner and Donor Attributes

## Owner Attributes

✓ It is important to select owners who are interested in the blood donor program and who understand that their pet's participation in the program truly saves lives. Conscientious owners will be helpful in monitoring the overall health status of the donor so that neither the blood donor nor the blood supply is compromised in any way.

## Donor Attributes

💣 Positive donor attributes can make the entire blood collection process easier for everyone involved. Potential donors should not bite or resist venipuncture or restraint. Blood donors should be of good disposition and good health.

### Physical Attributes

#### Canine Blood Donors

✓ Canine blood donors should weigh at least 50 pounds so that human blood collection bags (450-ml capacity) may be used. A maximum of 22 mL/kg of blood may be donated every 21 to 28 days; however, one donation every 3-4 months may be preferable to the owner.

✓ For ease of blood collection, donors should possess easily accessible jugular veins; there should be minimal neck folds or thick skin.

✓ The donor may be male or spayed nulliparous female.

✓ There should be no history of previous blood transfusions.

💣 Adherence to the above two criteria will eliminate donors who may have been exposed to foreign blood groups and could have potentially developed antibodies that may interfere with compatibility testing.

✔ Donors should be between 1 and 8 years of age.

✔ Vaccination status should be current and the donor should be on heartworm preventative.

✔ All coagulation factors including von Willebrand Factor levels should be normal.

## Feline Blood Donors

✔ Feline blood donors should be at least 10 pounds in weight. A maximum of 15 mL/kg can be drawn every 4 weeks; however, one donation every 3-4 months may be preferable to the owner.

✔ Although feline blood donors will most likely be sedated for phlebotomy, those with good dispositions should be chosen.

✔ An easily palatable jugular vein is desirable. A long neck and torso may contribute to ease of phlebotomy by providing a flat, smooth phlebotomy site.

✔ The donor may be male or spayed nulliparous female.

✔ There should be no history of previous blood transfusions.

♥ Adherence to the above two criteria will eliminate donors who may have been exposed to foreign blood groups and could have potentially developed antibodies that may interfere with compatibility testing.

✔ Donors should be between the ages of 1 and 8 years.

✔ To minimize exposure to feline infectious diseases, feline blood donors should be strictly indoor cats, with no exposure to outdoor cats.

✔ All coagulation factor levels should be normal.

# Laboratory Evaluation

✔ In addition to these physical traits, various laboratory tests should be performed to ensure the health status of the donor and to ensure the safety of the blood donor pool.

✔ For dogs, a complete hemogram and biochemical profile should be performed. Laboratory analysis for brucellosis, Lyme Disease, Rocky Mountain Spotted Fever, dirofilariasis, and Ehrlichiosis are recommended. Additional laboratory testing may be required to evaluate donor health status, including laboratory analysis to evaluate any disease endemic of the geographic locale.

✔ For cats, a complete hemogram and biochemical profile should be performed.  Laboratory analysis for feline leukemia virus, feline immunodeficiency virus, dirofilariasis and hemobartnellosis are recommended.  As with dogs, additional laboratory testing may be required to evaluate donor health status including laboratory analysis to evaluate any disease endemic of the geographic locale.

♥ One additional donor attribute to consider is the donor's blood type.  A brief discussion of canine and feline blood types in regard to donor selection follows.

## Canine

✔ Eleven canine blood groups have been described (Table 1-1).  More than one blood group can be present in any given donor.  Dog Erythrocyte Antigen (henceforth, "DEA") 1.1,1.2, and 7 are most important when considering canine blood transfusions.  DEA 1.1 and 1.2 are highly antigenic and previously sensitized dogs may have hemolytic transfusion reactions when transfused with DEA 1.1 or 1.2 blood.  If a transfusion of a random blood type is given, there is a 25% chance that DEA 1.1 or 1.2 positive blood will be given to a 1.1 or 1.2 negative dog.  Subsequent transfusions of the same offending blood type would result in major transfusion reaction s in at least 15% of these recipients.  DEA 7 is moderately antigenic to DEA 7 negative recipients.  This blood group may cause mild to moderate transfusion reactions and can decrease red cell survival when given to previously sensitized DEA 7 negative dogs.  Dogs that are DEA 1.1, 1.2, and 7 negative are considered universal donors.

✔ It is important to understand the significance of these blood types when selecting canine blood donors for a blood donor program.  The overall goal of the blood donor program should be considered.  If the majority of transfusions are expected to be a once-in-a-lifetime occurrence, the inclusion of all canine blood types may be appropriate.  This may assure a large number of donors for the program.  If most recipients are expected to need multiple transfusions, it may be appropriate to include only universal donors to the program in order to prohibit development of unexpected antibodies.

## Table 1-1 Canine Blood Group Frequencies

| System | DEA | Incidence | Additional Information |
|---|---|---|---|
| A | 1.1 | 45% in US | • Isoimmune antisera produced to one of the A antigens can cross-react with other antigens in the series<br>• If a DEA 1.1, 1.2, 1.3 negative dog is immunized with 1.3 positive cells, antisera strongly agglutinates and hemolyzes 1.1 and 1.2 positive cells and weakly reacts to 1.3 positive cells |
| | 1.2 | 20% in US | |
| | 1.3 | not evaluated in US | |
| | null | | |
| B | 3 | 6% in US | • Naturally occurring anti-DEA 3 occurs in 20% of DEA 3 neg dogs in US<br>• Transfusion of DEA 3 positive RC to sensitized dog = loss of transfused RC within 5 days and severe acute transfusion reaction |
| | null | | |
| C | 4 | 98% in US | • Naturally occurring anti-DEA 4 not reported<br>• DEA 4 negative dogs produce antibody when sensitized with DEA 4 positive red cells, but no RC loss or hemolysis when transfused |
| | null | | |
| 5 | 5 | | • Naturally occurring anti-DEA 5 in ~10% DEA 5 negative dogs in US<br>• Transfusion of DEA 5 positive red cells to sensitized dog = loss of transfused red cells within 3 days |
| | null | | |
| 6 | 6 | ~ 100% in US | • Naturally occurring anti-DEA 6 not reported<br><br>• Typing Sera no longer exists |
| | null | | |
| Tr | 7 (Tr) | 40-54% | • Naturally occurring anti-DEA 7 in 20-50% DEA 7 negative dogs<br>• If transfused to sensitized dog = loss of transfused red cells within 3 days<br>• Tr antigen is not RC membrane antigen, is produced and secreted in plasma and absorbed to RC |
| | 0 | | |
| | null | | |
| 8 | 8 | 40-45% | • Typing Sera no longer exists |

Other information on the A System:
• Anti-DEA 1.1 is a strong hemolysin in vivo and vitro
• Naturally occurring anti-DEA 1.1 and 1.2 have not been documented, so first time transfusion reactions should not occur
• Once sensitized, anti-DEA 1.1 and 1.2 can cause severe acute transfusion reaction with transfused red cells removed within 12 hours
• Transfusion of plasma with anti-DEA 1.1 to DEA 1.1 positive recipient causes hemolytic transfusion reaction
• DEA 1.2 positive recipient may produce strong anti-DEA 1.1 antibody when exposed to DEA 1.1 positive red cells. Immediate transfusion reaction can occur.

Condensed from: Feldman BF, Zinkl JG, Jain NC: Schalm's Veterinary Hematology, 5th Ed. Philadelphia, Lippincott Williams and Wilkins, 2000.

## Feline

✓ Three feline blood groups have been described (Table 1-2). They are A, B, and AB. Blood type A is the most frequent blood group, type B is much less frequent and type AB is extremely rare. Feline blood type frequencies differ in geographic location, as do the frequencies of type A and B in purebreds. It is important to note that cats do not need to be previously sensitized by pregnancy or previous transfusion in order to have serious complications from a first time transfusion. Unlike dogs, cats possess naturally occurring antibodies against the A or B antigen absent from their own red cells. These antibodies can be responsible for transfusion reactions and neonatal isoerythrolysis. With blood type B, 70% of cats have naturally occurring A antibody that causes decreased red cell survival and acute hemolysis when transfused to type A recipients. With type A, 35% of cats have naturally occurring B antibody; but the titer is generally too low to cause significant transfusion reactions. Type AB has no naturally occurring alloantibodies.

✓ When selecting feline blood donors for a blood donor program, blood type is extremely important. The blood type of the recipient population should be examined, and cats should be accepted to the program accordingly.

### Table 1-2  Feline Blood Group Frequencies

| | US GEOGRAPHIC LOCATION | | | | |
| BLOOD TYPE | SOUTHEAST | SOUTHWEST | NORTH CENTRAL | NORTHEAST | WEST COAST |
| --- | --- | --- | --- | --- | --- |
| A | 98.5% | 97.5% | 99.4% | 99.7% | 94.8% |
| B | 1.5% | 2.5% | 0.4% | 0.3% | 4.7% |
| AB | 0 | 0 | 0.2% | 0.0% | 0.5% |

Condensed from: Feldman BF, Zinkl JG, Jain NC: Schalm's Veterinary Hematology, 5th Ed. Philadelphia, Lippincott Williams and Wilkins, 2000.

# Donor Selection

✓ The criteria for selection of blood donors outlined above may be best evaluated at an office visit separate from a scheduled blood donation. This will provide the veterinarian time to evaluate physical exam findings and laboratory test results in view of the overall goals of the blood donor program. Once a donor is accepted into the blood donor program, this process should be repeated annually to maintain donor and product integrity. Donor blood types need not be checked on an annual basis.

# Keeping Track of Donors

✓ Once donors are qualified into the blood donor program, it is necessary to maintain information regarding individual donors in an easily accessible format. This may be done by creating a database that contains a variety of donor information including owner name, owner work and home phone numbers, donor medical record number, and last phlebotomy date. By performing this task, donors may be monitored for vaccination status, last annual check-up, and last phlebotomy date. This will be a valuable tool when scheduling donors for phlebotomy.

# Scheduling Donors for Phlebotomy

✓ Owners should be contacted to schedule phlebotomy in advance of the desired blood collection date. A consistent day and time (i.e., once every 8 weeks on Monday at 8 a.m.) for routine phlebotomy may be convenient for owners to remember their obligation to the blood donor program. However, if the phlebotomy is scheduled more than one week in advance, a reminder message may be necessary.

✓ When contacted for scheduling donation, owners should be asked about any change in the donor's health status since the last office visit or donation. A pre-phlebotomy questionnaire is helpful in accomplishing this task. This questionnaire should include any questions that may pertain to any change in health status such as recent weight loss, acute vomiting or diarrhea, or change in behavior. This questionnaire may be completed when contacting owners to schedule phlebotomy. This does not eliminate the need for a physical exam prior to blood donation.

# Basic Equipment Needs for Blood Collection, Processing, and Storage

## Blood Collection Bags

✓ Canine phlebotomies may be performed using human blood collection and storage bags. These are available through manufacturers listed in Appendix 1.

✓ Feline phlebotomies may be performed using a specialized blood collection and storage bag listed in Appendix 1. (Human blood collection and storage bags should NOT be used for cats.) Additionally, whole blood may be collected for immediate transfusion using an anticoagulated syringe; limited processing and storage occurs using this method of blood collection.

# For Canine Blood Collection

✓ A **vacuum chamber** (Figure 1-1) attached to a **vacuum source** can provide a light vacuum in which to facilitate blood flow into the blood collection bag.

✓ A **Tube Stripper** (Fenwal) is used to strip the blood out of the phlebotomy line  (Figure 1-2).

✓ A **Hand Sealer** (Fenwal) used in conjunction with metal clips will provide a method for sealing the lines of the blood collection bag.  Terumo's Hand Sealer and Aluminum Sealing Clip performs both functions  (Figure 1-3).  **Electric Heat Sealers** (Figure 1-4) are available from both manufacturers.

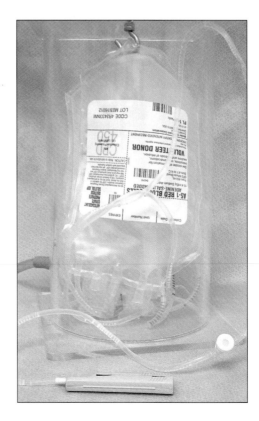

**Figure 1-1** Vacuum chamber.

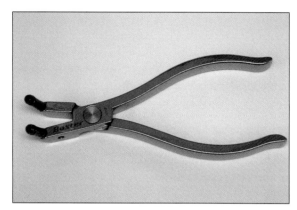

**Figure 1-2** Tube stripper. (Photo used with permission of Baxter Healthcare Corporation.)

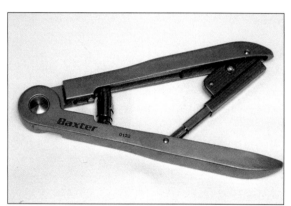

**Figure 1-3** Hand sealer. (Photo used with permission of Baxter Healthcare Corporation.)

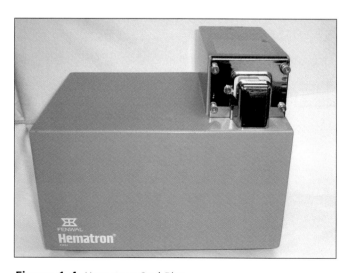

**Figure 1-4** Hematron Seal Rite.
(Photo used with permission of Baxter Healthcare Corporation.)

# For Whole Blood Separation

✓ In order to separate whole blood into red blood cells and fresh frozen plasma, a **refrigerated centrifuge** is needed. The necessary temperature range is 1-6° centigrade (C). A rotor head with swinging buckets will provide for maximum plasma recovery.

✓ A **Plasma Extractor** (Fenwal, Terumo) is needed for removing the appropriate quantity of plasma from the red cells (Figure 1-5).

✓ A **scale** for weighing products will be needed (Figure 1-6).

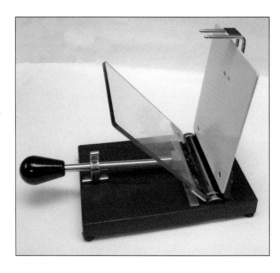

**Figure 1-5** Plasma extractor.
(Photo used with permission of Baxter Healthcare Corporation.)

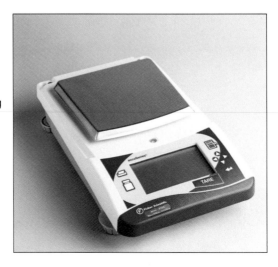

**Figure 1-6** Scale for weighing blood products.
(Image supplied by and used with permission of Fisher Scientific.)

# Blood Storage

✓ A **refrigerator** is needed to store red cell products. The temperature range should be from 1-6° C, with a method to monitor temperature.

✓ A **freezer** is needed to store frozen plasma products. These items should be stored at ⁻18° or below. A freezer dedicated to plasma storage is optimal. There should be some type of temperature monitor, be it human or electronic, to ensure that the product is stored at a constant temperature.

💣☀ Do not purchase a freezer with a defrost cycle since the defrost cycle may warm the product and cause unexpected degradation.

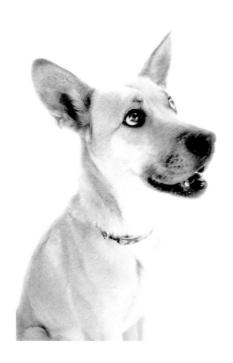

# Section 2

# Collection, Processing, Storage, and Shipment

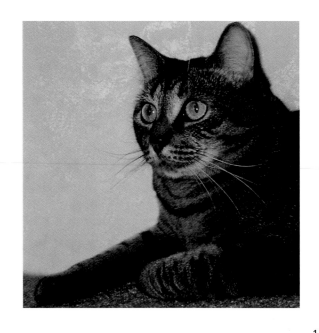

# Anticoagulants and Preservatives

✓ The following questions should be answered prior to blood collection and will assist in selecting the proper anticoagulant-preservative and blood collection system best suited to the product need.

What blood product is needed?
Will the product be used for immediate transfusion?
Will components be made?
Will the blood be stored?

## Anticoagulant-Preservatives

✓ Obviously, an anticoagulant should prevent coagulation of the unit of blood, thereby maintaining the unit in a liquid, trans-fusible state. However, the anticoagulant should also ensure that the blood product maintains its integrity so that the product will provide optimal benefit to the patient. Modern blood collection devices utilize a liquid solution that contains both anticoagulant **and** preservatives. The anticoagulant is citrate; the preservatives are phosphate-dextrose solutions. These solutions enhance preservation of the red cells and prevent detrimental changes to the product by maintaining pH and promoting adenosine triphosphate (ATP) production in order to maintain red cell viability. Citrate-phosphate-dextrose (CPD) and citrate-phos-phate-double-dextrose (CP2D) contain phosphate and dextrose. Citrate-phosphate-dextrose- adenine (CPDA1) has the addition of adenine to support red cell survival (Table 2-1).

✓ This combination of anticoagulant and preservatives provide an environment safe to store blood products: red cell products should be stored between 1-6° C, plasma products should be stored at ⁻18° C or lower. Platelets should be stored between 22-25° C.

✓ Anticoagulant-preservative solutions **do not** inhibit the growth of microbial contaminants. Refrigeration of red cells and freezing plasma products assists in inhibiting microbial growth within the blood product.

## Table 2-1 Anticoagulant-Preservatives/Additives Shelf Life

| ANTICOAGULANT | CONTAINS | RED CELL SHELF LIFE AT 1-6°C |
|---|---|---|
| Heparin | Heparin | 24 hours |

| ANTICOAGULANT-PRESERVATIVE | CONTAINS | RED CELL SHELF LIFE AT 1-6°C |
|---|---|---|
| ACD | Antigoagulant-citrate-dextrose | 21 days |
| CPD | Citrate-phosphate-dextrose | 21 days |
| CP2D | Citrate-phosphate-double-dextrose | 21 days |
| CPDA-1 | Citrate-phosphate-dextrose-adenine | 35 days |

| ADDITIVE | CONTAINS | RED CELL SHELF LIFE AT 1-6°C |
|---|---|---|
| AS-1 (Adsol®) | Dextrose, adenine, mannitol, sodium chloride | 42 days |
| AS-3 (Nutricel®) | Dextrose, adenine, monobasic sodium phosphate, sodium chloride sodium citate, citric acid | 42 days |
| AS-5 (Optisol®) | Dextrose, adenine, mannitol, sodium chloride | 42 days |

# Additives

✓ Like preservatives, additives are a combination of chemicals used to extend the life of the red cell. There are three commercially available additive solutions: Adsol® (AS-1, Fenwal), Nutricel® (AS-3, Haemonetics) and Optisol® (AS-5, Terumo). The constituents of these additives vary by manufacturer, but all contain dextrose, adenine, and sodium chloride. Other constituents that may be included are sodium phosphate, mannitol, sodium citrate, and citric acid.

✓ Additives are used **in addition to** anticoagulant-preservatives. The additive serves to increase red cell survival for a period of time **longer than** an anticoagulant-preservative alone. The additive allows for removal of maximal amounts of plasma from the unit of red cells. Since the additive solution is directly added to the red cells, the hematocrit of the unit of red cells is decreased, thereby creating a less viscous, more transfusible unit of blood. The additive must be added to the red blood cells within 72 hours of collection.

# Shelf Life

✓ Remember that a unit of blood is a biosystem and death is innate. The stored or "banked" product has a specific "shelf life." In general, shelf life is based on functional considerations in regard to blood components.

♥ The shelf life of a blood product is the maximum allowable storage time.

✓ The length of storage time is also affected by the nature of the blood collection device used: the device is "closed" or "open."

> ✓ A closed collection system does not allow its contents to be exposed to air or outside elements during collection, processing or storage.

>> ✓ Closed systems have integrally attached needles and satellite bags. The manufacturer places anticoagulant-preservative and additives in the system; these systems are available commercially. Use of a closed system promotes longer shelf life, which is dependent on the type of anticoagulant-preservative-additive used.

> ✓ An open system does expose its contents to air or outside elements at some point during collection, processing or storage. Use of an open system mandates the blood product be used within 4 hours if the product is stored between 22-25° C or 24 hours if stored at 1-6° C. Open systems include syringes and bags or bottles **without** integrally attached collection needles or satellite bags.

# Blood Collection Systems

## Canine Blood Collection Systems

### Open Systems

✓ As previously stated, open systems used in blood collection allows for blood to be exposed to air or outside elements at some point during collection, processing, or storage. This mandates that the product be used within 4 hours if stored at room temperature or 24 hours if stored at 1-6° C. Although many anticoagulants are available, some are better suited for blood collection and transfusion than others. Heparin and sodium citrate are two anticoagulants frequently used in open systems.

✓ Heparin acts as an anticoagulant by accelerating the action of antithrombin III, neutralizing thrombin, and preventing the formation of fibrin from fibrinogen. Heparin also deactivates platelets, making its use prohibitive for collection of blood for treatment of coagulation disorders. Heparin does not provide nutrients to facilitate red cell survival.

✓ Sodium citrate acts as an anticoagulant by chelating calcium. When used alone, sodium citrate is not suitable for collection of blood for transfusion due to its pH. Citrate used in conjunction with other chemicals is the anticoagulant of choice for collection of blood for transfusion because it has low toxicity and is easily metabolized. Glass bottles containing citrate dextrose (anticoagulant-citrate-dextrose, ACD) have been used in the veterinary field for many years. Since glass bottles are an open system, this product should be used within 24 hours of collection.

💣 Glass inactivates platelets, coagulation factor XII and factor VIII. Use of other blood collection systems may provide a superior blood product.

## Closed Systems

✓ A closed blood collection system does not allow blood to be exposed to air or outside elements during collection, processing or storage. Closed systems have integrally attached needles and satellite bags. In human blood collection systems (used for dogs), the manufacturer places anticoagulant-preservative and additives in the system (listed in Appendix 1). Anticoagulant must be added to the feline blood collection system (listed in Appendix 1).

✓ Anticoagulant-preservatives include ACD, CPD, CPDA-1, and CP2D. CPD and CPDA-1 are the most widely used in closed systems.

✓ ACD, CPD, or CP2D used in a closed system allows red cell shelf life of 21 days when stored at 1-6 degrees C, CPDA-1 allows red cell shelf life for up to 35 days when stored at 1-6 degrees C.

♥ Remember that blood bags purchased commercially have an expiration date independent of product collection. This expiration date guarantees anticoagulant-preservative activity and bag sterility.

## Additives

✓ Adsol® (AS-1, Fenwal), Nutricel® (AS-3, Haemonetics), and Optisol® (AS-5, Terumo) are three commercially available additives. These additives allow red cell shelf life of 42 days when stored at 1-6° C for 42 days. In human blood collection systems, these additives are used in conjunction with the anticoagulant CPD.

# Feline Blood Collection Systems

## Open Systems

✓ Remember that the volume of blood drawn from a feline donor is considerably less than that of its canine counterpart. A typical feline donation is approximately 50 milliliters, making 60 cc syringes a popular blood collection device for cats. Since this is an open system, blood stored at 1-6° C should be used within 24 hours of collection.

✓ The anticoagulant of choice is citrate phosphate dextrose adenine. The amount of blood taken into any citrate based anticoagulant is critical. Too little blood with too much free citrate is contraindicated for use in cats. Citrate not consumed in anticoagulation is a notable chelator of patient calcium, so much so that severe and often delayed hypocalcemia can occur. CPDA anticoagulant is far superior than any other commonly used anticoagulant as red cell viability is maintained and plasma proteins remain functional. This anticoagulant may be purchased from a commercial veterinary blood bank in multiuse vials.

## Closed Systems

✓ Blood collection systems used for canine blood collection are not suitable for collection of feline blood since the volume of anticoagulant in the blood collection bag used for canine is intended for a 450-ml blood draw. Although the amount of anticoagulant may be reduced in order to perform a smaller volume blood draw, the integrally attached 16-gage collection needle is too large for the feline jugular vein used to collect blood. For this reason, blood bags used for the collection of canine blood are not used with cats.

✓ A specialized blood collection system for cats (Figure 2-1) is available through Animal Blood Bank (Appendix 1).

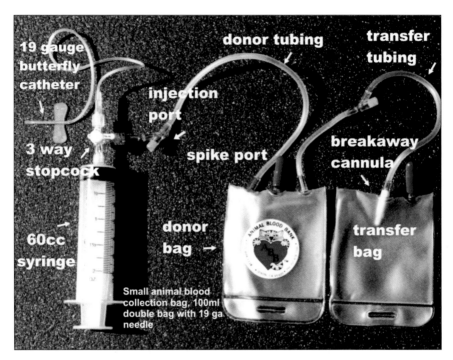

**Figure 2-1** Small animal double syringe collection set (Photo used with permission of Animal Blood Bank).

# Blood Product Overview

## Blood Products

✓ While the properties of blood products are similar in dogs and cats, this discussion is limited to closed systems and 450 ml blood draws.

♥ **Remember** – blood products collected in open systems should be transfused within 24 hours of collection. Closed systems **that have been opened** should be used within 24 hours of opening.

✓ The following information is summarized in Table 2-2.

## Table 2-2 Blood Product Overview

| PRODUCT NAME | CONTAINS | STORAGE | EXPIRATION |
|---|---|---|---|
| Fresh Whole Blood | All Blood Elements: Red Cells, Platelets Clotting Factors | 1-6° C | 24 hours |
| Whole Blood, Stored Whole Blood | Red Cells, Plasma Proteins, Stable Coagulation Factors | 1-6° C | ACD,CPD and CP2D: 21 Days CPDA-1: 35 Days |
| Red Blood Cells, Packed Cells | Red Blood Cells | 1-6° C | ACD,CPD and CP2D: 21 Days CPDA-1: 35 Days With Additive: 42 days |
| Fresh Frozen Plasma | All Coagulation Factors, Plasma Proteins | ⁻18° C or lower | 1 Year from Collection Date |
| Plasma | Vitamin K Dependent Factors, Albumin, Immunoglobulins | ⁻18° C or lower | 5 Years from Collection Date |
| Cryoprecipitated Antihemophilic Factor | Fibrinogen, Fibronectin, von Willebrand Factor, Factor VIII, XIII | ⁻18° C or lower | 1 Year from Collection Date |
| Cryoprecipate Poor Plasma | Fibrinogen, Fibronectin, Factors XI, XIII, VIII, von Willebrand Factor, Vitamin K Dependent Factors, Albumin, Globulins | ⁻18° C or lower | 1 Year from Collection Date |
| Platelet Rich Plasma | Platelets, All Coagulation Factors, Plasma Proteins | 22-25° C | Transfuse Immediately |

# Whole Blood and Red Cell Products

## Fresh Whole Blood

✔ Fresh whole blood provides blood volume expansion and increased oxygen carrying capacity to the recipient. It also delivers viable platelets and coagulation factors. It is often used for actively bleeding patients with acute blood volume loss of greater than 25%.

✔ A unit of whole blood is called fresh whole blood for a time period of 24 hours after phlebotomy.

✔ Fresh whole blood contains all blood elements: red cells, platelets, clotting factors and plasma proteins.

✔ Fresh whole blood is stored at 1-6° C.

✔ ACD, CPD, CP2D, and CPDA-1 are suitable anticoagulant-preservatives. The use of heparin is discouraged.

✔ Red cell additives are **NOT** mixed with whole blood.

✔ Due to its limited vitality, fresh whole blood is generally not available unless it is drawn immediately prior to its need. Since obtaining a blood donor on an emergency basis may not be practical, it may not be feasible to transfuse fresh whole blood. Instead, fresh whole blood is generally used for component preparation.

## Whole Blood and Stored Whole Blood

✓ Whole blood provides for volume expansion, increased oxygen carrying capacity, protein source, and stable coagulation factors.

✓ Once fresh whole blood is stored at 1-6° C for a period of time longer than 24 hours, it is called whole blood.

✓ Whole blood contains red cells and plasma proteins, but platelets and coagulation factors are diminished. Stable coagulation factors II, VII, IX, X, and fibrinogen are preserved.

✓ The anticoagulant-preservatives ACD, CPD, and CP2D maintain this product for 21 days. The use of CPDA-1 maintains whole blood for 35 days.

✓ Red cell additives are **NOT** mixed with whole blood.

✓ Storage of whole blood is an option for extending the use of a unit of fresh whole blood once the 24 hour shelf life is exceeded.

### Short draw

✓ Most commercially available blood bags are intended for a 450 ml + 45 ml blood volume. These bags contain 63 mls of anticoagulant-preservative for a final blood to anticoagulant ratio of 1:10.

✓ If 300-404 mls of blood is drawn into a bag intended for a 450 ml blood draw, the unit should be maintained as whole blood; components should not be made from this unit. The unit may be used for transfusion, but it should be labeled as a low volume unit. Underfilled units may cause citrate intoxication when transfused.

✓ If a blood collection of less than 300 mls of blood is needed, the amount of anticoagulant-preservative may be aseptically reduced prior to blood collection. (Please refer to page 39.)

## Red Blood Cells or Packed Cells

✓ Red blood cells assist in restoring oxygen carrying capacity to the recipient with less expansion of blood volume in comparison to whole blood. Red blood cells are used to treat anemia in normovolemic patients or pharmacologically untreatable anemia.

✓ Red blood cells are prepared from a unit of fresh whole blood or whole blood. To prepare this product, plasma is extracted from the unit of whole blood and the cells remaining in the bag are called red blood cells. This process may be expedited by centrifugation, or the red cells may be allowed to settle to the bottom of an undisturbed unit of whole blood. ACD, CPD, and CP2D provide a 21 day shelf life at 1-6° C. CPDA-1 provides for 35 day shelf life.

✓ Red cell additives will extend the life of a unit of red cells to 42 days at 1-6° C. Red blood cell additives must be mixed with red cells within 72 hours of phlebotomy.

# Plasma Products

## Fresh Frozen Plasma

✓ Fresh frozen plasma (FFP) contains all the coagulation factors, including the liable Factors V and VIII. It is a source of plasma proteins and volume expander. Fresh frozen plasma is used for treatment of patients with inadequate clotting factors for any reason. Fresh frozen plasma used in conjunction with red blood cells provide most of the benefits of fresh whole blood.

✓ Fresh frozen plasma is prepared from a unit of fresh whole blood. The plasma is separated from the red cells by centrifugation and removed. It is then completely frozen at -18° C or lower. Complete freezing of the plasma must occur within 8 hours of phlebotomy if the anticoagulant-preservative is CPD, CP2D, or CPDA-1. If ACD is used, separation and freezing must occur within 6 hours of phlebotomy. Once frozen, the product has a shelf life of 1 year from its original phlebotomy date.

## Plasma

✓ Plasma is used to treat stable clotting factor deficiencies. This product contains vitamin K dependent factors, albumin and immunoglobulins. It may be used as a volume expander, in warfarin/coumarin toxicity and canine parvovirus.

✓ This product is derived from extending the shelf life of a unit of fresh frozen plasma. When a unit of fresh frozen plasma is stored at -18° C in excess of one year, it is relabeled as Plasma. This is done to reflect the loss of clotting factors that occurs during the one-year storage.

✓ Plasma has a shelf life of 5 years from the original phlebotomy date. Plasma not separated from red blood cells within 6-8 hours after phlebotomy is labeled Plasma (**not** FFP.)

# Cryoprecipated Antihemophilic Factor

✓ Cryoprecipitated Antihemophilic Factor (AHF, also known as Cryoprecipitate or Cryo) is a rich source of VWF, Factor VIII, fibrinogen Factor XIII, and fibronectin. It is useful in the treatment of von Willebrand's Disease, Hemophilia A, hypofibrinogenenemia, disseminated intravascular coagulation, and septicemia.

✓ Cryoprecipitate is made from a unit of fresh frozen plasma. FFP contains high molecular weight plasma proteins which precipitate in the cold. When FFP is thawed at 1-6° C, the resulting precipitate is Cryoprecipitated AHF. After approximately 90% of the cryo poor plasma is removed, Cryoprecipitated AHF is refrozen and maintained at -18° C or lower. Its shelf life is for one year from the phlebotomy date.

# Cryoprecipitate Poor Plasma

✓ Cryoprecipitate Poor Plasma (Cryo-Poor Plasma) contains very low amounts of fibrinogen, fibronectin, Factors XI, XIII, VIII, and von Willebrand factor. It contains no Factor V. Cryo-poor plasma contains the vitamin K dependent factors, albumin and globulins. It is suitable treatment of canine parvovirus or coumarin/warfrin toxicity.

✓ Cryo-poor plasma is the residual plasma left from making cryo. When maintained at -18° C or lower, it has a shelf life of one year from the original phlebotomy date.

# Platelet Rich Plasma and Platelet Concentrates

✓ Platelets stop hemorrhage, as they are the first cellular element of the peripheral blood to react when blood vessels are damaged.

✓ Platelet Rich Plasma (PRP) is prepared by differential centrifugation from fresh whole blood that has been maintained between 22-25° C.

✓ In order to provide viable platelets to the recipient, platelet rich plasma should be transfused as soon as it is prepared.

✓ Platelet Concentrates are prepared by centrifugation of Platelet Rich Plasma. Excess plasma is removed and the remaining platelets are viable for at least 5 days from the phlebotomy date when stored between 22-25° C. In order to prevent platelet aggregation and to provide adequate oxygen and carbon dioxide exchange, platelet concentrates should be stored with gentle, continuous agitation.

# Blood Collection Systems and Pre-Processing Guidelines

## About Blood Collection Systems

✓ Blood Collection Systems are available in a variety of configurations. They are composed of the primary bag and satellite bags (Figure 2-2).

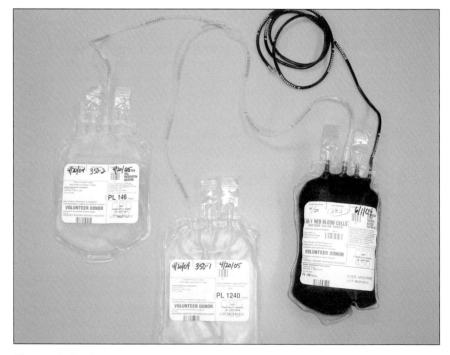

**Figure 2-2** Blood collection system (Photo used with permission of Baxter Healthcare Corporation.)

✓ The optimum blood draw volume is dependent on the Blood Collection System used. The draw volume is determined by the size of the bag and the amount of anticoagulant contained in the primary bag.

✓ The needle is attached to the primary bag. The primary bag contains anticoagulant; blood will flow directly into the primary bag during phlebotomy. Other smaller bags, which are integrally attached to the primary bag through sealed ports, are the satellite bags. There may be one or more satellite bags depending on the configuration of the blood collection system selected.

✓ Satellite bags intended for storage of red cells, plasma or platelets are labeled as such by the manufacturer.

# Pre-processing Guidelines

♥ All blood products should be labeled with the phlebotomy date, product name and expiration date. Additional information such as the blood type and donor may also be helpful. Permanent markers should be used for labeling so that this information is not washed off during storage, thawing or warming of the product.

✓ Before processing begins, the needle should be removed from the blood collection system. This is accomplished by heat seal (Hematron Dielectric Sealer, Baxter Healthcare, Fenwal Division) or metal clips (Hand Sealer, Hand Sealer Aluminum Clips, Baxter Healthcare, Fenwal Division.)

✓ Once the needle is removed, the phlebotomy line should be cleared using a tube stripper (Donor Tube Stripper, Baxter Healthcare, Fenwal Division). This will assure that the line is properly anticoagulated (Figure 2-3). This is important because this line will now be separated into segments (Figure 2-4) that will be used as the donor blood sample for compatibility testing.

✓ Each blood bag has a set of identification numbers repeated the length of the blood collection line. Place the first seal **after** the first identification number that is located at the top of the blood bag and repeat sealing segments for the length of the phlebotomy line. Fold segments end to end and rubber band them together. This will prevent the segments from getting tangled in the centrifuge head should the unit be processed for components (Figure 2-5).

✓ If segments are inadvertently separated from the blood bag during storage, the identification number on the segments can be compared to the identification number on the blood bag.

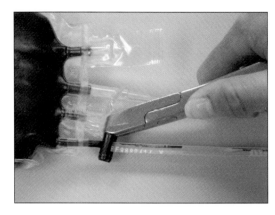

**Figure 2-3** Clearing the phlebotomy line.

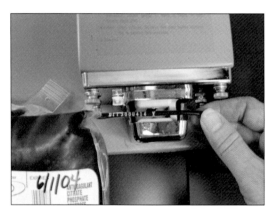

**Figure 2-4** Sealing the segments.

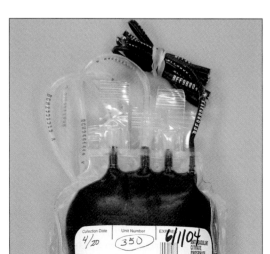

**Figure 2-5** Segments, secured.

# Preparation of Fresh Whole Blood

## Canine

✓ Once a unit of whole blood has been collected, it should be stored at 1-6° C until processing is possible unless it will be used to produce platelet preparations. A unit of whole blood is considered Fresh Whole Blood for a time period of 24 hours after phlebotomy. Fresh Whole Blood contains all blood elements.

✓ If absolutely no components will be processed from the unit of Fresh Whole Blood, the satellite bags may be sealed from the primary bag, detached and discarded.

✓ This procedure is repeated in a step-by-step format in the Methods Section.

## Feline

When a syringe or bag of feline whole blood is collected in an open system, it should be transfused as soon as possible. If significant delays are imminent, store the product at 1-6° C until transfusion is possible.

# Preparation of Red Cells and Fresh Frozen Plasma

✓ When the blood collection process is complete, the unit of whole blood should be stored at 1-6° C until component preparation is possible.

✓ This discussion is limited to 450 ml blood collection for dogs. For preparation of feline blood components, Animal Blood Bank (listed in Appendix 1) provides blood component preparation techniques with the purchase of the "Small Animal Double Syringe Collection Set."

✓ If the component Fresh Frozen Plasma is to be made, the plasma must be separated from the red cells and completely frozen within 8 hours of collection if the anticoagulant-preservative is CPD, CP2D, or CPDA-1. If the anticoagulant-preservative is ACD, separation and freezing must occur within 6 hours of phlebotomy.

✓ Whole blood designated for platelet preparations should remain at room temperature until the platelets are removed.

✓ This procedure is repeated in a step-by-step format in the Methods Section.

# Preparation for Centrifugation

✓ The entire unit of blood should be weighed. This weight is used exclusively for balancing the centrifuge.

✓ Proper centrifuge balance is important to prevent wear of the centrifuge rotor; total weight in opposing cups should be equal (Figure 2-6).

✓ An empty blood bag may be filled with 10% glycerin in order to provide an equally weighted balance bag for centrifugation. Rubber bands and weighted plastic discs may also be used to achieve balance (Figure 2-7).

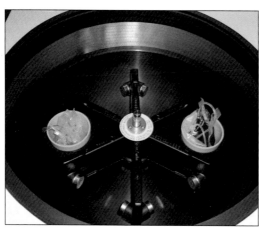

**Figure 2-6** A balanced centrifuge. (Photo used with permission of Kendro Laboratory Products.)

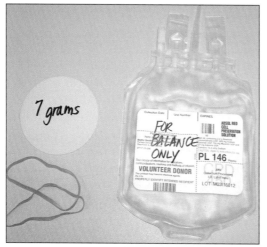

**Figure 2-7** Balancing devices.

# Centrifugation

✓ Blood bags should be placed in the centrifuge bucket with the label facing out. This reduces the centrifugal force on sealed margins of the blood bag. Centrifuges with swinging cups provide for easier separation of plasma from the red cells (Figure 2-6).

✓ The unit of whole blood should be centrifuged using a "heavy spin" in a refrigerated centrifuge between 1 and 6 degrees centigrade.

A heavy spin is defined as 5000 g for 5 minutes. (See "Centrifuge Calibration" in the Methods Section for further information regarding centrifuge speed and time.)

✓ Once centrifugation has ceased, it is important to allow the centrifuge to stop spinning without assistance, as brake use or an acute stop of the rotor will disturb the red cell/plasma separation, thus contaminating the plasma with red cells.

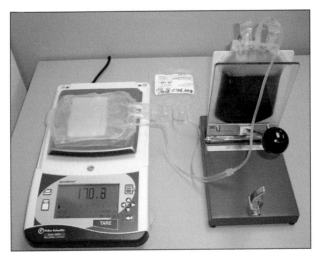

**Figure 2-8** Extracting plasma from centrifuged whole blood. (Image used with permission of Acculab and Baxter Healthcare Corporation.)

## Component Separation

✓ The unit of blood should be removed from the centrifuge without agitation so as not to disturb red cells and plasma. The unit should be placed on a plasma extractor (Fenwal; Plasma Separation Stand, Terumo®) This piece of equipment provides a rigid stand in which to place units of whole blood. A hinged plate is attached to the stand and may be released to apply pressure to the unit of whole blood in order to express the plasma into a satellite bag (see Figure 2-8).

♥ For this discussion, there are two satellite bags: one contains Adsol®, one is empty. However, the number of integrally attached satellite bags depends on the blood collection system being used.

✓ The plasma will be expressed into the empty satellite bag. The empty satellite bag should be placed on a balance. The weight should be tared to zero.

✓ Remove 230-256 grams of plasma.

**About this calculation:**

The specific gravity of plasma is 1.023, so 1 gram of plasma is approximately equal to 1 milliliter of plasma. Removing 230-256 grams of plasma will leave the unit of red cells with a final packed cell volume of 70-80%.

Note: This guideline should be followed using blood collection systems in which red cells will be supplemented with Adsol®. However, red cells may be prepared without Adsol® of varying packed cell volumes. See Table 2-3 for guidelines.

### Table 2-3 Preparation of Red Cells With Known Packed Cell Volume

|  |  | DONOR PCV | | |
|---|---|---|---|---|
|  |  | 35% | 40% | 45% |
| **DESIRED PCV** | 50% | 135 | 90 | 45 |
|  | 60% | 188 | 150 | 113 |
|  | 70% | 225 | 193 | 161 |
|  | 80% | 253 | 225 | 197 |

Shaded area denotes volume of plasma to be removed from 1 unit (450 mL) Whole Blood.
Volumes are approximate, based on 1gram = 1 mL

✓ Using hemostats, clamp off the line of the bag containing the harvested plasma. Then, break the seal from the Adsol® bag and let the Adsol® flow into the red cells. Seal the bag containing the red cells and Adsol® and remove the red cell bag from the plasma bags. Gently mix the red cells and Adsol®.

✓ Two satellite bags remain; one contains 230-256 grams of plasma with a volume of 225-250 mls. The plasma may be left in one bag, or divided equally between the two bags. Seal plasma bag(s) appropriately.

♥ The choice to divide the plasma should be made based on typical recipient size and plasma demand. Blood collection systems may be purchased with one to four satellite bags and should be selected accordingly.

✓ Tare the weight of the balance to zero and weigh each of the filled blood bags. The weight of the empty bag should be subtracted from the final weight of the bag. The specific gravity of red cells is 1.080-1.090; the specific gravity of plasma is 1.023. By dividing the final weight of the product by the appropriate specific gravity, the volume of product in milliliters can be calculated.

✓ The final product should be labeled with the product name and volume in milliliters. If Adsol® has been added to the red cells, this should be noted on the bag.

## Storage

✓ Red cells should be refrigerated at 1-6° C. While a refrigerator dedicated to blood storage is ideal, there are a variety of refrigerators available in a wide price range that maintain adequate temperature. The blood product should be stored in an organized fashion. It is advantageous to place the shortest date (the unit which expires first) at the front of the refrigerator so that it will be used first. Other products or supplies that may be stored in the same refrigerator should be segregated from the units of red cells (Figure 2-9).

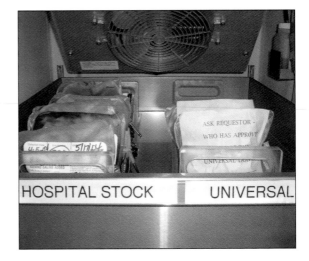

**Figure 2-9** Storage of red cells.

✓ Plasma products should be stored at ¯18° C or below. A freezer dedicated to plasma storage is optimal. Freezers used to store plasma products should not have a defrost cycle, since the defrost cycle may temporarily increase the temperature in the freezer and may cause inadvertent product thawing. Inadvertent product thawing may also occur during power outages.

✓ To monitor stored frozen plasma for inadvertent thawing, one of the two following techniques may be utilized (Figure 2-10).

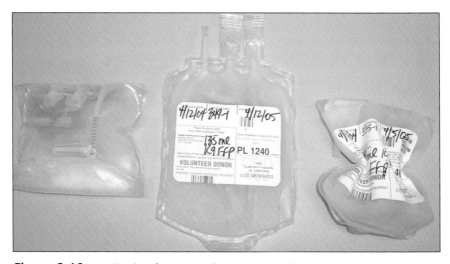

**Figure 2-10** Monitoring frozen product storage: The product on the right has a frozen "waist" indentation, while the product on the left contains dead space frozen at the bottom of the bag. The product in the center represents a product that has thawed and refrozen.

✓ A rubber band may be placed around the middle of a unit of plasma before it is frozen. Once the product freezes, the rubber band is removed, forming a "waist" indentation on the unit of plasma. If the unit thaws, the waist disappears. Thus, a unit of plasma removed from the freezer without the waist indention has likely been warmed above freezing during storage.

✓ Another technique that may be used involves initially freezing the unit of plasma inverted. This creates a "bubble" in the bottom of the plasma bag. Once frozen, the bag should be placed upright. Thus, if a unit of plasma is removed from the freezer without the bubble in the bottom of the bag, it has likely been warmed above freezing during storage.

✓ Additionally, an external temperature monitor on the plasma storage freezer(s) is helpful in monitoring freezer temperature. These monitors are available with electronic or chart readouts.

✓ Plastic blood storage bags may break if mishandled at temperatures below zero. To protect the frozen plasma, wrap the product in plastic bubble wrap prior to freezing. Frozen plasma products should be handled with care!

## Product Records

✓ A product log is helpful in tracking product use. Donor identification number, donation date, expiration date, volume of product, and final disposition of unit may be useful information to maintain.

# Preparation of Cryoprecipitated Anti-Hemophilic Factor and Cryo-Poor Plasma

✓ Cryoprecipitated Anti-Hemophilic Factor and Cryo-Poor Plasma are made from one unit of Fresh Frozen Plasma (FFP).

✓ To process Cryoprecipitated Anti-Hemophilic Factor from Fresh Frozen Plasma, a full unit (225-250 mL) of Fresh Frozen Plasma **with at least one integrally attached satellite bag** is needed.

✓ Fresh Frozen Plasma should be processed as outlined in the above procedure **except:**

✓ The **entire unit** (225-250 mL) of FFP should remain in one satellite bag.

It is important to document the total volume of the unit of FFP as this value will be used in a subsequent calculation.

✓ The line between the two satellite bags should be temporarily occluded in order to prevent transfer of plasma in to the second satellite bag.

✓ The FFP should be frozen solid before preparing Cryoprecipitated Anti-Hemophilic Factor.

✓ Allow the unit of Fresh Frozen Plasma to thaw at 1-6° C. This process takes approximately 8 hours. When the plasma has a slushy consistency, harvest the Cryoprecipitated Anti-Hemophilic Factor using one of the two following methods.

1. Place the thawing plasma in a plasma extractor. Express the liquid plasma into the empty integrally attached satellite bag. The newly filled satellite bag should contain 90% of the original volume of FFP. Seal both bags.

2. Centrifuge the plasma using a heavy spin. The Cryoprecipitated Anti-Hemophilic Factor will precipitate and adhere to the sides of the bag (Figure 2-11). Express 90% of the supernatant into the empty satellite bag. Seal both bags.

✓ The newly filled satellite bag containing 90% of the FFP is now Cryo-Poor Plasma. The satellite bag containing the residual 10% of the FFP is Cryoprecipitated Anti-Hemophilic Factor

✓ Freeze the Cryoprecipitated Anti-Hemophilic Factor and Cryo Poor Plasma within 1 hour of completion of preparation. Both products should be stored at ⁻18° C or lower.

✓ Product expiration is one year from the date of phlebotomy (not the date of preparation.)

✓ The product should be labeled with product name, total volume and expiration date.

✓ **This procedure is repeated in a step-by-step format in the Methods Section.**

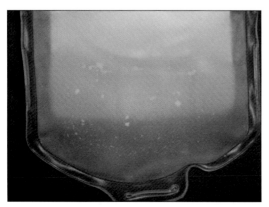

**Figure 2-11** Cryoprecipitate.

# Preparation of Platelet Rich Plasma

✓ Platelet Rich Plasma (PRP) is made from one unit of Fresh Whole Blood (450 ml draw).

✓ To prepare Platelet Rich Plasma, a unit of Fresh Whole Blood **with at least one integrally attached satellite bag is needed.** The unit of Fresh Whole Blood should be maintained at 22-25° C and processed immediately in order to harvest viable platelets.

## Preparation for Centrifugation

✓ The entire unit of blood should be weighed. This weight is used exclusively for balancing the centrifuge.

    ✓ Proper centrifuge balance is important to prevent wear of the centrifuge rotor; total weight in opposing cups should be equal (see Figure 2-6).

    ✓ An empty blood bag may be filled with 10% glycerin in order to provide an equally weighted balance bag for centrifugation. Rubber bands and weighted plastic discs may also be used to achieve balance (see Figure 2-7).

✓ The unit of whole blood should be centrifuged using a "light spin" in a refrigerated centrifuge between 22-25° C.

A light spin is defined as 2000 g for 3 minutes. (See "Centrifuge Calibration" in the Methods Section for further information regarding centrifuge speed and time.)

✓ Once centrifugation has ceased, it is important to allow the centrifuge to stop spinning without assistance, as brake use or an acute stop of the rotor will disturb the red cell/plasma separation, thus contaminating the plasma with red cells.

## Component Separation

✓ The unit of blood should be removed from the centrifuge without agitation so as not to disturb red cells and plasma. The unit should be placed on a plasma extractor (Fenwal; Plasma Separation Stand, Terumo®) This piece of equipment provides a rigid stand in which to place units of whole blood. A hinged plate is attached to the stand and may be released to apply pressure to the unit of whole blood in order to express the plasma into a satellite bag (see Figure 2-8).

✓ The plasma will be expressed into the empty satellite bag. The empty satellite bag should be placed on a balance. The weight should be tared to zero.

✓ Remove plasma.

💣 The task of extracting platelets from centrifuged whole blood can be challenging, as red cells lie just below the platelet layer (Figure 2-12). Platelet Rich Plasma should be light yellow in color and should not contain visible red cell contamination.

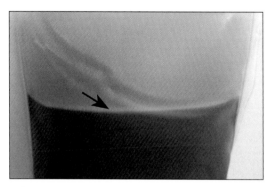

**Figure 2-12** Centrifuged fresh whole blood with platelet layer.

✓ Using hemostats, clamp off the line of the bag containing the harvested plasma and seal. Process the Red Cells as described on page 29.

✓ Calculate the volume of Platelet Rich Plasma.

*About this calculation:*

The specific gravity of plasma is 1.023, so 1 gram of plasma is approximately equal to 1 milliliter of plasma.

✓ Tare the weight of the balance to zero and weigh the Platelet Rich Plasma. The weight of the empty bag should be subtracted from the final weight of the bag. By dividing the final weight of the product by the appropriate specific gravity, the volume of product in milliliters can be calculated.

✓ The final product should be labeled with the product name and volume in milliliters.

## Storage

✓ In order to preserve platelet viability, Platelet Rich Plasma should be allowed to "rest" at room temperature, label side down for 1-2 hours and transfused as soon as possible thereafter.

✓ **This procedure is repeated in a step-by-step format in the Methods Section.**

# Short Draw and Decreasing the Amount of Anticoagulant-Preservative

✓ Commercially available blood bags are designed to anticoagulate and preserve a specific amount of blood. Deviations from the expected blood volume must be handled appropriately in order to assure product viability. This discussion will be limited to those bags designed for a 450 mL draw, although the principles may be applied to bags with a different expected draw volume.

## Short Draw

✓ Blood collection bags intended for a 450 mL draw contain approximately 63 mL of anticoagulant-preservative. This amount of anticoagulant-preservative is sufficient to support 405-495 mL of whole blood. If 300-404 mL of whole blood is drawn into a bag intended for a 450 mL draw, the unit of blood should not be processed into components and should remain as whole blood. The unit of blood should be labeled as "Short Draw" and the volume of the draw should be documented on the bag.

💣 Be aware that these units contain an increased amount of anticoagulant and citrate toxicity to the recipient is a concern. This may prohibit the use of short draw units of blood for some recipients.

## Decreasing the Amount of Anticoagulant-Preservative

✓ If a phlebotomy of less than 300 mL is planned, the amount of anticoagulant-preservative in the blood bag should be decreased prior to blood collection. Anticoagulant-preservative may be removed by expressing the excess anticoagulant-preservative solution into one of the integrally attached satellite bags.

✓ The calculation for the amount of anticoagulant-preservative to be removed:

Amount of Anticoagulant-Preservative needed in mL = (mL of Blood to be Drawn/100) X 14 mL Anticoagulant-Preservative to Remove from Primary Blood Bag = 63 mL – Amount of Anticoagulant-Preservative needed in mL.

💣☀ This calculation is valid only for anticoagulant-preservatives in which the ratio of anticoagulant to blood is 1.4:10. This includes most blood collection systems containing CPD or CPDA-1.

## Procedure for Removal of Anticoagulant-Preservative from Primary Blood Bag

✓ Obtain the specific gravity and amount of the anticoagulant-preservative in the primary bag. Calculate the weight of the anticoagulant-preservative to be removed from the primary bag.

✓ Weigh both the primary bag and the satellite bag designated for collection of excess anticoagulant-preservative.

✓ Open the seal from the primary bag. Express the calculated amount of anticoagulant-preservative to be removed into the empty satellite bag. Seal and remove the satellite bag.

✓ The unit may be processed for components.

# Purchasing and Receiving Blood Products from Outside Sources

## Purchasing Blood Products

✓ It may be necessary for a veterinary practice to order blood products from outside sources.

• This could be due to an emergency case that consumes all stored blood products during a time period of which donors are not readily available for blood donation.

• Some veterinary practices may order blood products from outside sources exclusively.

✓ A veterinary blood bank should be identified.

• Some veterinary blood banks that provide blood products for purchase are listed in Appendix 2.

- It is advisable to establish a client relationship with the blood supplier before the need for blood products arises.

✓ Communication regarding anticipated need of blood products provides the supplier with valuable information; the supplier can adjust blood collection so that adequate blood supplies may be maintained.

- This also provides the purchaser an opportunity to inquire as to methods of collection and quality of the donor pool.

- Additionally, the purchaser may obtain information regarding the suppliers policies and procedures regarding ordering blood products.  Caveat emptor!

✓ The purchaser might inquire:

- What is the purchase price of the product?

- How long does it usually take to get product on a routine basis?

- How long will it take to obtain the product on an emergency basis?

- How will the product be packed?

- Once packed, how long does the packing permit the product optimal storage temperatures?

- Will overnight shipping be used? What are the associated costs?

- Does the delivery route incur extremely hot or extremely cold outside temperatures?  Will the packing materials compensate for this?

- Are temperature monitoring devices used for the shipping process?  Time temperature tags, high-low thermometers (Taylor Instruments, Rochester, NY) or R&D Temperature Indicators (Chek Lab Inc, Aurora, IL) may be used.

- What is the policy if units are received that have exceeded acceptable shipping temperatures?

- What is the policy if the unit is mishandled or lost during shipping?

- What will the expiration date(s) of the unit(s) be?

# Receiving Blood Products

✓ Upon receipt of the product, immediately unpack the product.

✓ Perform a visual inspection. Is the product damaged in any way? Is there any leaking?

✓ Does it appear that the product has been maintained at the proper temperature?

- If no temperature monitoring device is used, the temperature of Red Cells may be checked by folding the blood bag in half (labels facing out) and wedge a thermometer within the "sandwich" of the bag (Figure 2-13). Read the temperature; it should not exceed 10° C.

- Frozen products should arrive frozen!

✓ The product should be placed at appropriate storage temperature and documented as received in the product log.

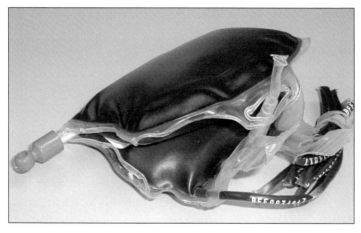

**Figure 2-13** Acquiring red cell temperature by "sandwich" technique.

# Preparing Blood Products for Shipment

✓ Blood products should be packaged and shipped in a manner that preserves product integrity.

💣 Federal, state, and local guidelines should be reviewed. In some instances, it is necessary to obtain licensure from federal or state agencies prior to shipping blood products.

# Product Packaging

✓ Transport containers and packaging procedures should be validated prior to use. These protocols should be periodically monitored to ensure the proper product temperature is maintained throughout the shipping process.

✓ Transport containers should have tight fitting covers and withstand leakage and pressure. Most shippers require that a cooler be shipped with a cardboard box cover. Address labels should be inscribed legibly with indelible ink.

✓ To package blood products for shipping:

1. Obtain a suitable transport container.
2. Within the container, starting from the bottom, layer:

   Coolant

   Absorbent paper

   Product

   Absorbent paper

   Coolant

   Container lid

3. Secure the coolant lid and exterior box.
4. Attach label.
5. Deliver to shipper.

✓ For Whole Blood and Red Cells, the coolant of choice is ice, which may be confined in a zippered closure plastic bag.

✓ For frozen products, dry ice is the coolant of choice.

💣 Dry ice is considered a hazardous material as it causes skin burns and releases carbon dioxide as it volatizes. Be sure to notify the shipper that the package contains this hazardous material.

✓ Absorbent paper should be capable of containing any leakage within the package. Paper towels, newsprint or disposable diapers are suitable.

✓ The blood product should also be secured in a zippered closure plastic bag in case of accidental damage resulting in subsequent product leakage.

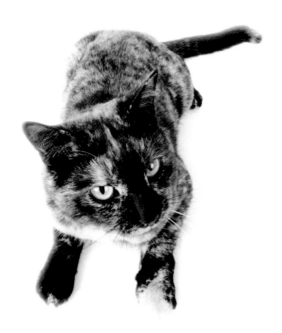

# Section 3

# Clinical Considerations in Transfusion Practice

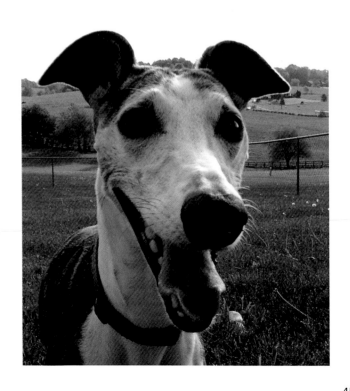

# The Crossmatch

The major and minor crossmatch are performed to assist in providing compatible red cell products and possibly alleviating adverse reactions to transfusion.

✓ The major crossmatch is performed to detect antibodies in the recipient's serum that may agglutinate or lyse the donor's erythrocytes.

✓ Conversely, the minor crossmatch detects antibodies in the donor plasma directed against recipient erythrocytes.

## About the Minor Crossmatch

✓ The minor crossmatch test procedure mixes the red cells of the recipient with the plasma from the donor. After appropriate incubation, the cell/plasma mixture is centrifuged and observed for agglutination. This test was widely used in human medicine until the advent of antibody screening cells. The advent of antibody screening cells to donor blood screening protocols eliminated the need for the minor crossmatch.

What are antibody screening cells?

Antibody screening cells are commercially available red cells that are human blood type O. These cells have been tested for common clinically significant human blood group antigens (such as the Rh system, MNS, Lewis, P, Kell, and others.) Antibody screening cells are typically sold in sets consisting of three antigentically different red cell samples. When used in human medicine for donor screening protocols, the plasma of a blood donor is tested against a set of antibody screening cells. If the antibody screen is negative, it can be assumed that the blood from the donor being tested is free from antibodies to the human blood group antigens present on the antibody screening cells. If the antibody screen is positive, another panel of screening cells is tested against the donor plasma and the antibody is identified. Remember that whole blood is separated into components and a positive antibody screen and identification may only exclude the donor plasma from the donor pool for routine transfusion. If the antibody screen is negative, it is assumed that the plasma can be safely transfused to an ABO compatible recipient. It is for this reason that routinely there is no crossmatch performed on plasma products in human medicine.

So what about veterinary medicine?

Currently, antibody screening cells are not available for veterinary use. **This is why the minor crossmatch is so important.** Remember that in the minor crossmatch, the red cells of the recipient are tested with plasma from the donor. This testing is performed to provide a safe transfusion, especially in the case that whole blood or plasma is used. In addition, think of the minor crossmatch in regard to the donor screening process: recipient red cells are acting as anti body screening cells. Indeed, these cells may or may not contain clinically significant antigens. But when a particular donor is tested against one or more samples of recipient red cells through the use of the minor crossmatch and found to be negative, a very general assumption can be made that there are no clinically significant antibodies in the donor plasma. Keep in mind that most blood donors will be qualified into a blood donor program for a time period of at least one year. It follows that there could be at least 4 blood donations per year with donor plasma being tested against at least one sample of recipient red cells for each donation. If the blood donor program is willing to accept this as a method of antibody screening donors, then it follows that plasma products may be transfused without a minor cross match being performed.

✓ Concurrently, it is advantageous to reject potential donors from the blood donor program who have been previously sensitized to foreign red cell antigens. This assists in eliminating plasma from the blood donor pool that potentially carries antibodies to red cell antigens.

# Blood Transfusion Guidelines

## Rationale for Therapy

Whole blood is a mixture of cellular constituents suspended in a liquid transport medium. The cells have different functions. Erythrocytes carry oxygen and participate in host defense by surface adsorption and absorption of many materials, phagocytes control bacteria, platelets are required for hemostasis, and lymphocytes mediate immunity. The liquid medium also contains an array of dissolved substances: albumin, globulins, coagulation proteins, metabolic intermediates, electrolytes, organic anions, and trace elements. Practical techniques for separation and concentration of some of the cellular constituents of whole blood are within the capabilities of all major veterinary blood donor centers. Modern transfusion therapy should be based upon use of components to treat specific defects with concentrates of the deficient blood constituent. There are a number of rationales for the preferential use of blood components.

# Consideration of the Limited Resource

The most cogent argument supporting component therapy is that blood is a precious resource considering its therapeutic potential and the logistics and costs required in obtaining and delivering blood products. Separation into components permits a single donation to meet the individual needs of more than several patients. Blood donor screening eligibility criteria should be sufficient to obtain a safe donation.

# Kinetic Considerations

Following hemorrhage, homeostatic mechanisms restore the various blood constituents at differing rates, depending on the capacity for synthesis, endogenous consumption, degradation, and distribution in various physiologic compartments. The half-inactivation time of canine and feline red cells is in terms of months whereas the half-life of albumin is just three to four days. Surgical blood loss may require restoration of red cells. Albumin may not be required, as it will be restored within several days. Another consideration is tolerance. Loss of 50% of red cell mass is well tolerated in a healthy individual whereas loss of 50% of blood volume can be fatal unless rapidly corrected.

# Consideration of Adverse Effects

Other rationale for supporting the use of blood components include the myriad of possible adverse effects that can result from transfusion of unnecessary blood constituents. Any transfusion reaction means that the transfusion is not performing the intended job and, importantly, has burdened a patient already burdened by the physiologic state requiring transfusion. Sensitization to blood cells can result in refractory results in subsequent transfusions. Transfusion of multiple units of whole blood sequentially in order to achieve a certain hematocrit may also produce pulmonary edema due to volume overload.

# The Decision to Transfuse

All transfusion therapy can produce only transient improvement in the patient's condition. Unless the patient is able to produce the deficit component endogenously, more transfusions will be necessary. Furthermore, transfusions dampen the physiologic response to deficiency of a blood constituent. For example, if a patient has a low red cell mass, tissue hypoxia results in increased erythropoietin production and the marrow responds with reticulocytosis. Red cell transfusion, in this patient, will result in diminished and delayed reticulocyte response. Several questions should be considered prior to transfusion.

> Is blood transfusion really necessary?
> What is the patient's particular need?
> Does the prospective benefit justify the risks of transfusion?
> What blood component will effectively meet this special need at the lowest cost?
> After transfusion:  Did the transfusion result in the anticipated benefit for the patient?

Answers to these questions should be documented in the patient's record. As a minimum for red cell transfusion, a pre-transfusion hematocrit and total protein should be followed by posttransfusion (24 hour) determinations.

Blood components may be conveniently classified according to their physiologic functions: oxygen transport, as an adjunct in intravascular volume maintenance, hemostasis and phagocytosis. In veterinary medicine, support of phagocytosis with granulocyte transfusions has not been accomplished. Volume replacement requires maintenance of colloid oncotic pressure (COP) through the use of colloids (hetastarch, pentastarch, dextrans, gelatin products) in addition to plasma. Albumin administered in the form of plasma to hypooncotic (hypoalbuminemic) patients not receiving concurrent colloidal support will rapidly equilibrate with third spaces.

# Transfusion to Increase Oxygen Transport

There is no set hemoglobin or hematocrit concentration below which a patient needs red cells. Patients and patient care dictate when red cells are required. A patient who has lost one third of his red cell mass acutely will require increased oxygen carrying capacity. Patients with chronic processes may have dramatically low hematocrits and, if not stressed, not require additional oxygen carrying capacity. However, in general terms, in both the dog and the cat, administering red cells to meet oxygen transport needs should be considered when hemoglobin concentration is below 7 grams per deciliter (hematocrit of 21%). When considering transfusion in specific patients, the clinician should consider age, etiology and duration of anemia, presence of coexisting cardiac, pulmonary, or vascular conditions, and hemodynamic stability.

# Products Which Increase Oxygen Transport

Whole Blood – Acute massive blood loss exceeding 20% of blood volume (appropriate blood volume is 90 mL/kg-canine, 70 mL/kg-feline), coagulopathy with massive blood loss, the hematocrit will increase over the baseline value immediately after transfusion and increase further within 24 hours with volume redistribution.

Red Cells (RC, Packed Cells) – RC are achieved when refrigerated whole blood is centrifuged in refrigeration and the plasma is removed. Because the hematocrit will approximate 70-80%, RC are often mixed with sterile saline or with an additive solution do decrease viscosity.

To determine the anticipated hematocrit in patients receiving red cells, calculate total blood volume (see Whole Blood above) and the total volume of the red cells (calculated from the pre-transfusion hematocrit). Determine the total blood volume after administering the transfusion (pretransfusion blood volume + volume of transfusion). Determine the new hematocrit by adding the volume of transfused red cells to the pretransfusion red cell volume. Anticipated post-transfusion hematocrit is the post-transfusion red cell volume divided by the post-transfusion total blood volume.

# Blood Substitutes: Alternatives to Blood and Blood Products

## Red Blood Cell Substitutes

Requirements for a successful red blood cell substitute:

1. It must work
2. Have a long shelf life
3. Be minimally immunogenic
4. Be pathogen and endotoxin free
5. Be readily available at a reasonable cost
6. Must deliver and release oxygen to tissues under clinical conditions

Clinical indications for a red blood cell substitute:

1. Acute anemia
2. Acute blood loss
3. Preoperative therapy
4. Intraoperative replacement
5. Useful to provide oxygen as a radiosensitizer in treatment of neoplasia

Hemoglobin based solutions:

Hemoglobin based oxygen-carrying solutions are a form of blood substitute used to increase the oxygen content of blood and improve oxygen delivery to tissues. Hemoglobin is carried in plasma. Hemoglobin in plasma increases the efficiency of offloading oxygen from blood cells to tissues by facilitating diffusion of oxygen through the plasma. Hemoglobin based solutions have long storage life and are useful immediately. These solutions are polymerized stroma-free hemoglobin which are virtually free of red cell membranes and as such are minimally immunogenic. These solutions deliver and release oxygen for 18 to 24 hours. There are effects on laboratory tests but effects are generally known, predicted, or minimal. These changes depend on the instrument used. Serum urea nitrogen and electrolytes appear to be unaffected. Administration of these solutions turns mucous membranes yellow to red to brown for at least several days.

Characteristics of a hemoglobin based oxygen-carrying solution approved for use in dogs (Oxyglobin® Solution) Biopure Corporation, Cambridge, Massachusetts)

This product has a physiologic hemoglobin concentration of 13 g/dL and is delivered in isosmotic lactated Ringer's solution. The average molecular weight of this solution is 200kD with a range of 65-500 kD . In this solution the oxygen affinity is dependent upon chloride ions. This is in contrast to red cell oxygen delivery which is dependent upon 2.3-diphosphoglycerate (2,3-DPG). The solutions are universally compatible and are stable at room temperature.

Indications for use – Oxyglobin® is useful in treating anemia due to any cause including hemolysis, blood loss due to trauma, surgery, gastrointestinal or genitourinary hemorrhage, or rodenticide toxicity causing hemorrhage.

Adminmistration and monitoring – The rate of delivery of Oxyglobin® is $\leq$ 10 mL/kg/hour in normovolemic canine patients. The signs of improved oxygenation include stabilization of vital signs such as heart and respiratory rates. Of course, the underlying cause of anemia must be treated. Mucous membranes and sclerae may transiently become yellow to red or brown. Volume expansion must be monitored. Decreases in red cell mass (packed cell volume; hematocrit) are predicted due to hemodilution. However, hemoglobin concentration rises.

Effects of low colloid oncotic pressure – noncardiogenic pulmonary edema, generalized edema, hypovolemia.

# Plasma Substitutes

Hetastarch as a plasma expander – This is a synthetic polymer (a waxy starch amylopectin) produced by DuPont Pharmaceuticals under the name Hespan®. It is six percent hetastarch in normal (0.9%) saline which almost iso-osmotic (310 mOsm/L). Hespan has a twelve-month shelf life. Administration dosages vary depending on authors. Twenty-five mLs/kg has a 7.5-8.4 day half inactivation time.

Safety and side effects – Hetastarch has low toxicity in humans and dogs. In nonoliguric renal failure renal function may improve. There are no apparent effects on granulocyte function. Hemostasis may be significantly affected. Platelet numbers and function may be reduced. The prothrombin (PT) and activated partial thromboplastin times (APTT) may be prolonged. Anaphylactic reactions have been reported.

Advantages of colloid (hetastarch) therapy – Colloid oncotic pressure (COP) I s improved. There is expansion of plasma volume without increase in interstitial water content. The use of hetastarch compares well with albumin and dextran containing solutions. It is safe for acute and long term usage. Single injections can increase plasma volume and COP for greater than forty-eight hours.

Hetastarch is useful in hypoalbuminemic dogs and cats. Current dosage recommendations are 30-35 mLs/kg/day with repeat usage depending on clinical judgement.

Contraindications of hetastarch – Hetastarch is contraindicated in cardiac insufficiency and in oliguric renal failure. Hetastarch is contraindicated in hemorrhage due to von Willebrand's disease and may be contraindicated when hemostasis is compromised or may be compromised.

VetaPlasma® (Smith Kline Beecham)

VetaPlasma® is marketed as a colloidal plasma expander (**it is NOT plasma**) in a physiologic electrolyte solution with a pH of 7.4. It is for intravenous use in dogs and cats. VetaPlasma® is oxypolygelatin with an average molecular weight of 30,000 Daltons. It does not increase plasma viscosity. It may improve renal function but it is excreted primarily (88%) though the kidneys. Vetaplasma® may cause anaphylactoid reactions. It has a relatively short half inactivation time (2-4 hours) and is hypoosmotic (200 mOsm/L). There is minimal (but some) hemostatic dysfunction with use of this product.

# Compatible IV Solutions

✓ 0.9% sodium chloride injection may be used to facilitate infusion of blood products.

✓ No medications or any other solution should be added to blood products unless the product is approved by the US FDA or there is adequate documentation that the product is safe for use with blood products.

✓ Various intravenous solutions interfere with blood transfusion.

• Lactated ringer's solution contains enough calcium to overcome chelating agents in anticoagulant-preservative additive systems. This results clot formation in the infusion line.

• 5% dextrose in water causes red cells to clump in the infusion line, causing red cells to swell and hemolyze.

# Blood Administration Sets

✓ Blood administration sets are used for the infusion of blood products.

✓ The use of a blood administration set assists in preventing potentially dangerous artifacts from being infused to the recipient. These sets contain a filter that serves to retain clots and other microaggregate particles that form in stored blood. The size of the particle retained by the filter is directly related to the size of the filter.

✓ Blood administration sets should be used with all blood components including platelet concentrates. Deviations from the manufacturer's instructions should be avoided as this may render the blood product ineffective. For example, using the inappropriate administration set for the infusion of platelet products could cause platelets to be inappropriately retained within the infusion set, defeating the purpose of transfusion.

✓ There are a variety of infusion sets commercially available. The manufacturer should be consulted regarding suggested use.

💣 Remember: any blood set should be changed every 4 hours. This is due to the fact that overt bacterial contamination may occur after longer periods of time.

✓ Some blood administration sets are designed for transfusion of more than one unit of blood, but total use time should not exceed four hours.

✓ Blood administration sets should not be reused due to the threat of bacterial contamination.

✓ There are two types of Blood Administration Sets: Gravity Drip and Syringe Push.

  ✓ Gravity Drip

  Standard blood administration sets contain a filter with a pore size of 170-260 microns. The set should be primed according to the manufacturer's directions with blood or blood-compatible fluid. For optimal flow rate, the filter should be fully wet and the drip chamber should be no more than half full during transfusion. Standard sets are typically used to transfuse whole blood, red cells, and plasma products. As the name implies, this set is attached to the blood product and the blood product is infused by gravity drip.

✓ Syringe Push

Syringe push sets may be used for component infusion or in the transfusion of products with a volume of less than 100 mls. This blood administration set uses the smallest priming volume of all sets. These sets have a smaller drip chamber and shorter tubing length than gravity infusion sets. This is helpful in the transfusion of small volume products. Syringe push sets contain an in-line filter that is extremely small and it may go unnoticed.

Blood products may be transfused in one of two ways using this infusion set. This set may be attached to a blood bag, the product drawn in to the attached syringe. The product is then "pushed" into the recipient. Alternately, this set may be attached directly to a syringe of blood for immediate transfusion. This may be useful in the transfusion of feline whole blood.

# Adverse Effects of Blood Transfusion

✓ The basic principle in transfusion therapy is the same as in all medical approaches, "primum non nocere" – first do no harm. Though transfusion fatality rate is small, deaths do occur, especially in cats, and morbidity varies significantly between institutions. Hemolytic reactions can be the most serious problem. Careful observation of clinical signs and appropriate laboratory evaluation of adverse effects of transfusion result in safe transfusion practices.

## Signs of Transfusion Reactions

✓ Febrile or allergic reactions may occur with fever or chills in the same manner as severe hemolytic reaction. For this reason, any adverse change in the patient's condition should be considered a possible sign of adverse transfusion reaction and should be evaluated.

✓ The essential elements that should take place when a transfusion reaction is suspected are:

1. Stop the transfusion.

2. The intravenous access should be kept patent for treatment if necessary.

3. The responsible clinician must be notified to evaluate the patient.

✓ Individuals who have had multiple transfusion or who have had prior pregnancies are at greatest risk for febrile reactions. A patient who has had a febrile reaction is a greater risk for subsequent reactions. Premedication does not appear be markedly effective in these cases and does not eliminate the need for astute observation.

✓ When a reaction is suspected, the administration set should be changed. This allows the 10-15 mls of blood remaining in the tubing to be discarded rather than infused in the patient.

# Complication—Immediate Immnologic Effects

## Hemolytic Reactions

Hemolytic reactions are most severe but are rare and are due to incompatible blood or intradonor incompatibility in multiple transfusions. Because cats have naturally occurring alloanti bodies in plasma (in particular, strong anti-A in type B cats), feline donor and recipient should be blood typed and cross matched prior to the transfusion. Feline AB mis-matched transfusions are ineffective and may cause life-threatening hemolytic transfusion reactions.

💣 It should be noted that hemolysis can be a nonimmunologic problem. Hemolysis usually results from physical destruction of cells by overheating or mixing nonisotonic solutions with red cells. **NO OTHER solutions should be infused through the transfusion site unless the transfusion is complete.**

### Signs

Chills (shaking), fever, pain at needle site or along venous tract, nausea, vomiting, darkened urine, flank pain, and if progressive, signs of shock and/or renal failure.

### Precautions

✓ If possible, identify donor and recipient blood types before transfusion is initiated. Perform compatibility testing.

✓ Transfuse blood slowly for first 15-20 minutes and/or initial 20% of the anticipated transfusion volume; remain with patient during this period.

### Response

✓ In the event of a reaction:

- Stop the transfusion.
- Maintain intravenous line.
- Notify the clinician.
- Save donor blood to re-crossmatch with the patient's blood.

✓ If possible:

- Monitor blood pressure for shock.
- Insert urinary catheter and monitor outputs hourly.
- Send sample of patient's blood and urine to the laboratory. Hemoglobinuria indicates intravascular hemolysis.
- Observe for signs of hemorrhage resulting from disseminated intravascular coagulation (DIC).
- Support therapies to reverse shock.

## Febrile Reactions

Any increase of one degree (Celsius) or more must be considered a febrile reaction due to white cell, platelet or plasma protein antibodies.

### Signs

Fever, chills

### Precautions/Response

✓ Stop the transfusion immediately.

✓ Consider antiallergy therapy.

## Allergic Reactions

Patient reacts to allergens in donor blood-red cells, platelets, granulocytes, plasma proteins-often complement-immunoglobulins.

### Signs

Urticaria, dyspnea, laryngeal edema

### Precautions/Response

✓ Give antiallergy therapy for prophylaxis in patients with allergic tendencies, although this is often ineffective.

✔ Stop the transfusion immediately.

✔ Epinephrine may be used for dyspnea or anaphylactic reaction.

# Complication—Immediate Nonimmunologic Effects

## Circulatory Overload

Circulatory overload is due to too rapid transfusion (even small quantities) or excessive quantity of blood (even if administered slowly).

### Signs

Dyspnea, rales, cyanosis, dry cough, distended neck veins (if visible, may be palpable).

### Precautions/Response

✔ Transfuse blood slowly.

✔ Prevent overload by using red cells or administering divided amounts of blood.

✔ Use an infusion pump to regulate and maintain flow rate.

✔ If signs of overload appear, stop the transfusion immediately.

## Hypothermia

Hypothermia is most often initiated by administering chilled blood product too rapidly.

### Signs

Chills, lowering temperature, irregular heart rate, possible cardiac arrest

### Precautions/Response

✔ Use a warming device to warm the blood product.

✔ If patient exhibits chills (shaking) and if patient body temperature is subnormal (from baseline), stop the transfusion.

## Electrolyte Disturbances

Electrolyte disturbances are rare but are often associated with patients with renal compromise.

### Signs

Nausea, diarrhea, muscular weakness, flaccid paralysis, bradycardia, apprehension, cardiac arrest

### Precautions/Response

✓ Use saline washed red cells or fresh whole blood for patients at risk.

## Citrate Intoxication (Hypocalcemia)

Citrate intoxication occurs especially in cats and with the use products which contain excessive anticoagulant due to short draws.

### Signs

Tetany, muscular cramps, hyperactive reflexes, seizure activity, laryngeal spasm, respiratory arrest

### Precautions/Response

✓ Infuse blood slowly.

✓ If tetany occur, clamp infusion tubing immediately, maintain patent intravenous line, notify clinician.

# Complication—Delayed Immunologic Effects

## Delayed Hemolytic Reaction

### Signs

Destruction of red cells and fever 10 to 15 days after transfusion. This is often and anamnestic response.

### Precautions/Response

✓ Observe for post-transfusion anemia and decreasing benefit from successive transfusions.

## Graft vs. Host

Graft vs. host is a rare complication following transfusion to severely  immunosuppressed patients such as those being intensively treated for immune-mediated disease, or being immunosuppressed with chemotherapy or radiation.  Graft vs. host occurs if immunocompetent donor lymphocytes engraft and multiply in immunodeficient patient.  Engrafted donor cells react against "foreign" cells of host-recipient.

### Signs

Fever, sking rash, hepatitis, diarrhea, bone marrow suppression

### Precautions/Response

✓ In human medicine, blood products may be irradiated. Red cell, granulocyte and platelet function are unaffected. Eighty-five to 95% of lymphocytes are rendered incapable of replication.

✓ Treatment is supportive and symptomatic.

# Post-transfusion Purpura

Post-transfusion purpura is a rare development if antiplatelet antibody. Post-transfusion purpura occurs most exclusively in multiparous dogs (rarely cats).

### Signs

Petechiae, purpura, ecchymosis follow precipitous fall in platelet count about one week post-transfusion. The antibody destroys both transfused and native platelets.

### Precautions/Response

✓ Immunosuppressive therapy

✓ If life threatening, in human medicine, plasma exchange is initiated.

✓ The problem is often self limiting in dogs.

# Alloimmunization (Antibody Formation)

Patient reacts to allergens in donor blood–red cells, platelets, granulocytes, plasma proteins–often complement–immunoglobulins.

### Signs

Increased risk of hemolytic, febrile and allergic reactions

### Precautions/Response

✓ Occurs in patients receiving multiple transfusions. Thus, transfuse products from a limited number of donors and observe patient for signs of reaction.

# Complication—Delayed Nonimmunologic Effects

## Transmission of Infection

### Signs

Icterus from hepatitis, fever, nonspecific discomfort or pain (often around chest wall or sternum), hypotension, vomiting, diarrhea

### Precautions/Response

✓ Query blood bank for anything notable currently associated with donor.

✓ Educate owners as to potential infectious signs.

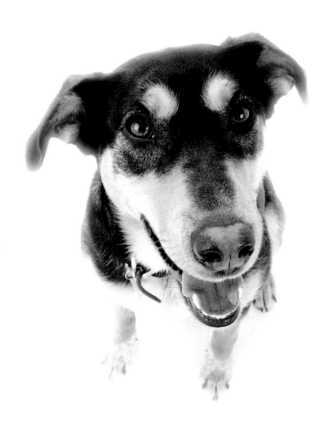

# Section 4

# Biosafety

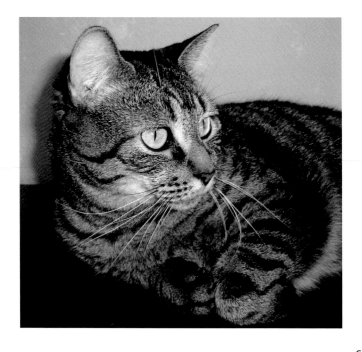

# Laboratory Safety

✓ It is the responsibility of every employer to provide a safe work environment for employees. This may be accomplished by developing and implementing a safety plan for the workplace. The goal of the safety plan should be to protect employees from situations that may compromise their health and well being. Although the development of the safety plan may be a tedious task, it is well worth the effort. The following is a **general** discussion for development of a safety plan. In addition, federal, state, and local guidelines should be consulted and followed.

✓ The safety plan should include a fire plan, accident plan, chemical plan, and maintenance of Material Safety Data Sheets (MSDS.) Other plans and policies should be added according to activities performed at the workplace. The safety plan should encompass all hazards found at the workplace.

✓ The fire plan should include a policy of what is expected of the employee in the case of a fire, including emergency telephone number(s). This policy should explain if the employee should fight the fire and at what point employee and patient evacuation is necessary. It is a good idea to assign employees to assemble at a specific area outside the work area so that employees may be accounted for. Employees should be trained in all areas of fire safety including location and use of fire extinguishers.

✓ The accident plan should include policies and procedures regarding on the job accidents. Minor and extremely serious accidents can occur on the job and every accident should be reported to the employer within 24 hours of its' occurrence. An accident report form may be helpful in documentation of accidents and necessary follow-up. It may be beneficial to specify in the accident plan the name and phone number of the physician with whom the injured employee should consult, if necessary.

✓ A chemical plan should include a list of all hazardous chemicals found in the workplace. The chemical plan should include a policy for secondary labels. Secondary labels are placed on containers of chemicals that have been removed from their original or primary containers. For example, if isopropyl alcohol is poured from it's original container into another container, it should be labeled with a secondary label. The secondary label should contain the product name, the preparation date or transfer date, and any necessary hazard information, such as "Eye Irritant."

✓ In conjunction with the chemical plan, Material Safety Data Sheets (MSDS) should be maintained for all chemicals listed on the chemical inventory. These sheets are supplied by the manufacturer, and are generally shipped with a product that is considered hazardous. For some household items, the manufacturer may need to be contacted in order to obtain the MSDS. The MSDS contain helpful information including but not limited to hazardous ingredients, physical and chemical information, fire and explosion data, health hazard data and precautions for handling. This information contained in the MSDS is useful in case of accidental spills, splashes, or inadvertent injection or ingestion.

✓ Other issues that necessitate safety policies and procedures include disposal of hazardous material, sharps and biohazards. A separate policy may be needed for each of these items. It may be beneficial to include in the biohazard policy exactly how expired blood components should be disposed of.

✓ The employer may want to supply a stocked first aid cabinet for employees. An Eye Wash Station should be available in case of inadvertent splashes in the eye. Protective clothing and equipment should be furnished by the employer and a policy regarding its' use. A policy on handwashing may also be beneficial.

✓ Ergonomic workstations and furniture may help prevent employee back problems. There are multitudes of manufacturers available for consultation.

✓ Once the appropriate safety policies and procedures are formulated and documented, it is important to provide safety training for each employee. There should be a form or worksheet to document this training. This training should be continual and ongoing as products used and work assignments change.

# Quality Assurance

## What is Quality Assurance?

✓ Quality assurance is a philosophy of the work place that provides an organization with information to examine and regulate the quality of patient care. Examining issues related to quality assurance may assist the organization in setting high standards of patient care through constant improvement of service. This may be accomplished by setting goals regarding quality assurance. All aspects of patient care may be analyzed and monitored; the challenge is to regulate variables therein.

✓ For a Blood Bank or Transfusion Service, the main goal of a quality assurance program should be to provide a safe transfusion for every patient.

# How is This Best Accomplished?

✓ First, it is advantageous to establish a committee of staff members to serve on a quality assurance team. The team should define and set goals related to quality assurance. While the quality assurance team may examine quality issues of an entire organization, this discussion will be limited to issues related to the Blood Bank or Transfusion Service.

   • As previously discussed, the organization should have safety policies and procedures in place. In addition, practical and concise policy and procedure manuals should be available for every task performed in the Transfusion Service. These procedure manuals should provide employees with a detailed outline for performance of a given task.

✓ The main purpose of a quality assurance team may be to identify and monitor quality indicators. Quality indicators can be devised to analyze work tasks that may be measured or monitored in some manner. Obtaining or improving the task measurement may improve the service.

   • For example, one of the quality indicators for the Blood Bank may be to monitor the length of time it takes to draw one 450-ml unit of blood. The American Association of Blood Banks specifies a target time of 4-10 minutes for a 450-ml phlebotomy. The quality assurance team may include this time specification in the phlebotomy procedure. The staff who perform the canine phlebotomies can use this as a benchmark for optimal draw time.

✓ Other quality indicators may include one or more of the following:

   • Check donors for bruising around the phlebotomy site. Excessive bruising may indicate the need for variation phlebotomy technique.

   • Survey donor owners as to their satisfaction in regard to the blood donor program. Owners who are satisfied with the care given to their animals are more likely to continue in the blood donor program and recommend the program to their friends.

✓ Periodic review of product labels for component type, phlebotomy date, expiration date, and donor identification.

✓ Periodic review of product inventory and use.

✓ Quality control on blood components. Products near or beyond expiration date may be used to monitor preparation techniques.

• For example, the hematocrit of expired Red Cells may be examined to verify that the designated final packed cell volume has been reached. Variation may indicate a problem in component preparation.

✓ Performing blood cultures on expired Red Cells may verify that aseptic phlebotomy and component preparation has occurred.

✓ Cryoprecipitate may be analyzed for Factor VIII and fibrinogen activity periodically to ensure that component preparation is optimal.

✓ Review of all transfusion reactions. Is there any common occurrence with transfusions that result in adverse reactions?

✓ Review of accidents related to products such as broken blood bags or contaminated ports.

✓ Review of equipment checks and temperature checks of refrigerators, freezers, water baths and blood warmers.

✓ Other quality indicators may be formulated as needed.

# Records

✓ Records provide a method of communicating with others regarding documentation of information including observations and opinions. This chapter will discuss several different types of records that may be used in a veterinary Blood Bank or Transfusion Service. Guidelines for documentation, maintenance and storage of these records will be discussed. Additionally, federal, state and local guidelines should be consulted and followed.

# What Attributes are Needed to Produce a Record of Good Quality?

✓ A record should be legible and accurate.

✓ It should include the transcription date and identity of the author.

✓ The record should make sense, be complete and as detailed as necessary to convey meaning.

✓ The record should also be indelible.

For a Blood Bank or Transfusion Service, records are typically inscribed by paper or computer. While the attributes listed above pertain to both paper and computer records, there are a few additional items regarding computer records that deserve mentioning.

> ✓ Computer records should be validated for accuracy.

> ✓ The system and data should be backed up regularly.

> ✓ Data should be protected from unauthorized access and inadvertent changes.

# Specific Records Related to the Blood Bank

✓ A Blood Bank or Transfusion Service should maintain certain records pertaining to blood donors and blood recipients.

> 💣 Failure to maintain these records on blood donors could endanger the blood supply, since valuable information regarding donor health status at the time of donation could be forgotten or lost.

✓ Guidelines for the maintenance of these records follow.

## Donor Records

Donor records should be composed of:

✓ Initial screening including physical exam findings, laboratory results, vaccination status, heartworm medication

✓ Consent form signed by the owner

✓ Physical Exam prior to each blood donation

✓ Annual Recheck including physical exam findings, laboratory results, vaccination status, heartworm medication

✓ Documentation of any follow up, if necessary

## Records Related to the Blood Bank Laboratory

The Blood Bank may perform laboratory testing in addition to donor testing. Items pertinent to the Blood Bank laboratory that should be retained are:

- ✔ Blood storage refrigerator and freezer temperature charts
- ✔ Equipment maintenance records
- ✔ Reagent vendors
- ✔ Quality Control of reagents
- ✔ Quality Control of donor units
- ✔ Blood typing and crossmatching results
- ✔ Transfusion records

✔ In regard to blood and blood components, a donor log composed of the date the unit of blood was collected, the unit identification, final volume, expiration date, identification of the preparer and the final disposition of the unit of blood should be maintained.

✔ If blood products are acquired from an outside source, the log should include these units.

- • Pertinent information includes who the products were purchased from, the date they were received, the name and identification of the component and expiration date.

## Record Storage: How Long?

✔ Remember: Records are stored over a period of time for investigative and legal purposes. Federal, state and local guidelines should be consulted and followed. If there are no guidelines, it may be helpful to store laboratory records for at least 2 years and medical records indefinitely.

# Inventory Management

✔ Blood product inventory management is difficult since use of blood products can be unpredictable and erratic. Blood products are a valuable commodity and every effort should be made to utilize this product efficiently. It is beneficial to devise a plan for the management of blood products so that this valuable resource is used in a timely and efficient manner.

✓ First, the optimal number of stored units of blood components should be established. **Each** stored product should be analyzed to determine the desired inventory level for that product. If specific blood groups of a particular product are needed, each blood group should be analyzed separately.

- For a 6-month period, collect data of product usage.
- Disregard any unusually high values of use.
- Total the number of units.
- Divide by the total number of weeks the data are collected.

The value generated from this analysis is the optimum stock level of product per week.

✓ Other factors should also be considered when determining optimal stock levels of blood product.

- The number of patients serviced by the veterinary practice. A high number of patients potentially need a high number of products. Endemic disease and accident rates should be considered.

- The size of the area serviced by the hospital. A large service area could result in a large number of patients who may need transfusions.

- The average weight of the recipient. What size dogs are popular within the service area? Large dogs may use more product than small dogs.

- The expiration date of the product. Which anticoagulant-preservative-additive system is used? If product is received from a supplier, what is the average expiration date?

- Services offered at the veterinary practice. An emergency clinic will use more blood products than a clinic that offers only routine services.

✓ It may also be useful to institute internal policies in regard to blood products to assist in inventory management. These policies should be communicated every staff member who may transfuse blood products.

> ✓ Use the oldest unit first. Arrange the refrigerator and so that the oldest unit will be pulled first. This will make using the oldest unit **convenient**.

> ✓ Institute ordering guidelines. Make sure each clinician knows that once the order is given to transfuse, the component will be warmed and the product **must** be used.

✓ Institute guidelines for issuing blood components. Specify how many units may be prepared for one patient at a given time. It may be appropriate to warm only one unit for one patient at a time, depending on the clinical situation.

What if products are not stocked, such as the case of feline whole blood?

✓ The number of blood donors needed should be calculated.

✓ Use the formula for calculating optimal stock level above.

• In addition to the list of "Other Factors," consider the frequency that blood may be obtained from a particular blood donor.

• The resulting value will provide an estimate of the approximate number of feline blood donors needed for the blood donor program.

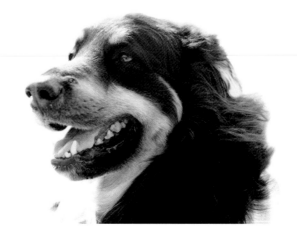

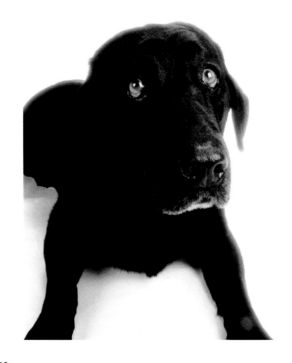

# Section 5
# Methods

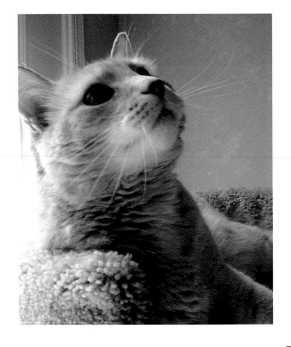

# Preparation of Fresh Whole Blood

## Canine

✓ Once a unit of whole blood has been collected, it should be stored at 1-6° C until processing is possible.

✓ A unit of whole blood is considered Fresh Whole blood for a time period of 24 hours after phlebotomy.

✓ Fresh Whole Blood contains all blood elements.

### Preparation of Fresh Whole Blood

1. To begin processing the unit of blood, restrip the line in which the needle was formerly attached. This will ensure that this line is adequately anticoagulated. This step is important because this line will now be sealed into segments that will later be used as the donor blood sample for compatibility testing.

Each blood bag has a set of identification numbers on the blood collection line. Place the first seal **after** the identification number that is located at the top of the blood bag, beside the ports (see Figure 2-4). That way, if segments are inadvertently separated from the blood bag during storage, the segments can be compared to the blood bag to confirm identification.

2. Fold the segments end to end and rubber band them together (see Figure 2-5).

3. If absolutely no components will be made from this unit of Fresh Whole Blood, seal off the satellite bags and discard them.

✓ If **Plasma** will be harvested more than 6 hours after phlebotomy, leave the satellite bags attached.

💣 Note: If the component **Fresh Frozen Plasma** is to be made, the plasma must be separated from the red cells and completely frozen within 8 hours of collection if the anticoagulant-preservative is CPD, CP2D or CPDA-1. If the anticoagulant- preservative is ACD, separation and freezing must occur within 6 hours of phlebotomy.

**Plasma** may be harvested at any time during the shelf life of the unit.

4. Label the product with the product name, volume of product and expiration date.

5. Fresh Whole Blood should be refrigerated between 1-6° C.

   ✓ Whole blood designated for platelet preparations should remain at room temperature until the platelets are removed.

## Feline

✓ When a syringe of whole blood is collected, it should be transfused as soon as possible.

✓ If significant delays are imminent, store the product at 1-6° C until transfusion is possible.

✓ When using the Small Animal Double Syringe Collection Set, please consult the directions supplied by Animal Blood Bank.

# Preparation of Red Cells and Fresh Frozen Plasma

## Canine

✓ Once a unit of whole blood has been collected, it should be stored at 1-6° C until component preparation is possible.

✓ If the component Fresh Frozen Plasma is to be made, the plasma must be separated from the red cells and completely frozen within 8 hours of collection if the anticoagulant-preservative is CPD, CP2D, or CPDA-1. If the anticoagulant- preservative is ACD, separation and freezing must occur within 6 hours of phlebotomy.

✓ Whole blood used for preparation of platelet components should remain at room temperature until the platelets are removed.

### Separation of Red Cells and Plasma

#### Preparation for Centrifugation

1. To begin the process of component preparation, restrip the line in which the needle was formerly attached. This will ensure the line is adequately anticoagulated. This step is important because this line will now be divided into segments that will later be used as the donor blood sample for compatibility testing.

Each blood bag has identifying numbers on the blood collection line. Place the first seal **after** the first identification number that is located at the top of the blood bag, beside the ports (see Figure 2-4). That way, if segments are inadvertently separated from the blood bag during storage, the segments can be compared to the blood bag to confirm identification.

2. Fold the segments end to end and rubber band them together (see Figure 2-5). This will assist in preventing the segments from getting tangled in the centrifuge head during blood processing.

3. The bag containing the whole blood should be labeled with the donor number. This is a good time to add the collection date and expiration date to the bag of whole blood.

💣 Expiration dates are determined by the type of anticoagulant and preservative used. Table 2-1 contains expiration date guidelines.

The satellite bag(s) should also be labeled with the component name, collection date, donor number and expiration date.

💣 Permanent markers should be used so that numbers will not be washed off during storage, warming or thawing.

4. The entire unit of blood and attached satellite bags should be weighed. This weight is used exclusively for balancing the centrifuge.

• Proper centrifuge balancing is important for wear of the centrifuge rotor; total weight in opposing cups should be equal.

• When processing an odd number of whole blood units, centrifuge balance may be achieved by using blood collection bags filled with an equal weight of 10% glycerin.

• Rubber bands and weighted plastic discs may be used to vary weight increments.

## Centrifugation

5. Blood bags should be placed in centrifuge cups with the label facing out. The centrifuge cups should be placed in the centrifuge with the bag label facing out. This reduces the centrifugal force on sealed margins.

✓ Centrifuges with swinging cups provide for easier separation of plasma from the red cells.

6.  The unit of whole blood should be centrifuged using a heavy spin in a refrigerated centrifuge between 1-6° C.  A heavy spin is defined as 5000 g for 5 minutes.  (See "Centrifuge Calibration" in this section for more information regarding centrifuge speed and time.)

💣 Once centrifugation has ceased, it is important to allow the centrifuge to stop spinning without operator intervention; any acute stop of the rotor, including brake use, will disturb the red cell/plasma line thereby contaminating the plasma with red cells.

## Component Separation

7.  The unit of whole blood should be removed from the centrifuge without agitation so as not to disturb red cells and plasma and placed on a plasma extractor (Fenwal; Plasma Separation Stand, Terumo®.)

✓ The plasma extractor provides a rigid stand in which to place units of whole blood.  A hinged plate is attached to the stand and may be released to apply pressure to the unit of whole blood in order to express the plasma into a satellite bag (see Figure 2-8).

8.  One empty satellite bag should be placed on a balance.  The weight should be tared to zero.  The plasma will be expressed into the empty satellite bag.

♥ The number of integrally attached satellite bags is dependent on the blood collection system being used.  For this discussion, a triple bag is used: there are two satellite bags, one contains Adsol®, one is empty.

9.  Open the plastic port at the top of the blood collection bag.  Remove 230-256 grams of plasma by releasing the hinged plate of the plasma extractor and applying pressure to the bag containing the centrifuged whole blood.  Plasma will be expressed into the empty satellite bag.

✓ The specific gravity of plasma is 1.023.  Therefore, removing 230-256 grams of plasma will leave the unit of red cells with a final hematocrit of 70-80%.

♥ Red cells may be prepared of varying packed cell volume, see Table 2-3 for guidelines.

10.  Once the desired plasma weight is achieved, use hemostats to clamp off the line of the bag containing the harvested plasma.  Then, break the seal from the Adsol®

bag and let the Adsol® flow into the bag that contains the red cells. Seal and detach the bag containing the red cells and Adsol® from the plasma bags. Gently mix the red cells and Adsol®.

## Plasma Separation

11. Two satellite bags remain; one contains 230-256 grams of plasma with a volume of 225-250 mls. The plasma may be left in one bag, or divided equally between the two bags.

♥ Final plasma bag volume should be based on typical recipient size and plasma availability.

Seal plasma bag(s).

## Determine Volume

12. The final volume of the blood product is determined as follows.

• Tare the weight of the balance to zero. Weigh each of the filled blood bags.

• The weight of the empty bag is subtracted from the final weight of the blood product. The final weight of the product divided by its specific gravity equals the volume of product in milliliters.

• The specific gravity of red cells is 1.080-1.090; the specific gravity of plasma is 1.023.

13. The blood product should be labeled with the product name and volume in milliliters.

♥ If Adsol® has been added to the red cells, this should be noted on the bag.

## Storage

14. Red Cells should be refrigerated between 1-6° C. Fresh Frozen Plasma should be stored at ⁻18° C or lower.

# Feline

✓ For preparation of feline blood components, Animal Blood Bank (listed in Appendix 1) provides blood component preparation techniques with the purchase of the Small Animal Double Syringe Collection Set.

# Preparation of Cryoprecipitate and Cryoprecipitate-Poor Plasma

## Canine

✓ Cryoprecipitated Antihemophilic Factor (AHF, also known as Cryoprecipitate or Cryo) is made from one unit (225-250 mls) of Fresh Frozen Plasma.

✓ Cryo is the insoluble portion of plasma that precipitates when a unit of Fresh Frozen Plasma is thawed between 1-6° C. The excess plasma is removed from the precipitate, creating Cryoprecipitate Poor Plasma (Cryo-Poor Plasma.)

✓ To make Cryoprecipitate, a full unit (225-250 mls) of Fresh Frozen Plasma **with at least one integrally attached satellite bag** is needed.

• When harvesting the Fresh Frozen Plasma from the unit of Whole Blood, allow the plasma to flow into one satellite bag. Seal off the two bags, but leave the line between the two bags open.

• Freeze the unit of plasma as specified in the procedure for Fresh Frozen Plasma.

• The plasma must be frozen solid before the subsequent steps to make cryoprecipitate are carried out.

### Separation of Cryoprecipitate and Cryoprecipitate-Poor Plasma

✓ Allow the unit of Fresh Frozen Plasma to thaw at 1-6° C. This process takes approximately 8 hours.

1. Harvest the cryoprecipitate using one of the two following methods:

✓ When the plasma becomes slushy, place the thawed plasma in a plasma extractor. Express the liquid plasma in to the integrally attached satellite bag. The satellite bag containing liquid plasma should contain 90% of the original volume of the Fresh Frozen Plasma.

OR

✓ Allow the Fresh Frozen Plasma to completely thaw. Centrifuge the FFP using a heavy spin. The cryoprecipitate will precipitate and adhere to the sides of the bag (see Figure 2-11). Express 90% of the supernatant in to the attached satellite bag.

Using either method, the Cryoprecipitate Poor Plasma is expressed into the satellite bag and the Cryoprecipitate remains in the bag that originally held the Fresh Frozen Plasma.

2. Seal both bags.

3. Determine the final volume. Label the product with the product name, final volume and expiration date.

💣 Product expiration is one year from the date of phlebotomy (**not** from the date of preparation.)

## Storage

4. Freeze the Cryoprecipitate and the Cryo Poor Plasma within 1 hour of preparation. Both products should be stored at ⁻18° C or lower.

**NOTE:**

As an alternative, Cryoprecipitate may be prepared from stocked FFP by allowing the FFP to thaw (as outlined above) and removing the Cryo-Poor Plasma using a syringe. As this creates an "open" environment, the product should be used within 24 hours of preparation.

# Preparation of Platelet Rich Plasma

✓ Platelet Rich Plasma is made from one unit of Fresh Whole Blood.

✓ To prepare Platelet Rich Plasma, a unit of Fresh Whole Blood **with at least one integrally attached satellite bag** is needed. The unit of Fresh Whole Blood should be maintained at 22-25° C and processed immediately in order to harvest viable platelets.

# Separation of Red Cells and Platelet Rich Plasma

## Preparation for Centrifugation

1. To begin the process of component preparation, re-strip the line in which the needle was formerly attached. This will ensure the line is adequately anticoagulated. This step is important because this line will now be divided into segments that will later be used as the donor blood sample for compatibility testing.

Each blood bag has identifying numbers on the blood collection line. Place the first seal **after** the first identification number that is located at the top of the blood bag, beside the ports (see Figure 2-4). That way, if segments are inadvertently separated from the blood bag during storage, the segments can be compared to the blood bag to confirm identification.

2. Fold the segments end to end and rubber band them together (see Figure 2-5). This will assist in preventing the segments from getting tangled in the centrifuge head during blood processing.

3. The bag containing the whole blood should be labeled with the donor number. This is a good time to add the collection date and expiration date to the bag of whole blood.

💣 Expiration dates are determined by the type of anticoagulant and preservative used. Table 2-1 contains expiration date guidelines.

The satellite bag(s) should also be labeled with the component name, collection date, donor number and expiration date.

💣 Permanent markers should be used so that numbers will not be washed off during storage, warming or thawing.

4. The entire unit of blood and attached satellite bags should be weighed. This weight is used exclusively for balancing the centrifuge.

✓ Proper centrifuge balancing is important for wear of the centrifuge rotor; total weight in opposing cups should be equal.

✓ When processing an odd number of whole blood units, centrifuge balance may be achieved by using blood collection bags filled with an equal weight of 10% glycerin.

✓ Rubber bands and weighted plastic discs may be used to vary weight increments.

# Centrifugation

5. Blood bags should be placed in centrifuge cups with the label facing out. The centrifuge cups should be placed in the centrifuge with the bag label facing out. This reduces the centrifugal force on sealed margins.

✓ Centrifuges with swinging cups provide for easier separation of plasma from the red cells.

6. The unit of whole blood should be centrifuged using a light spin in a centrifuge between 22-25° C. A light spin is defined as 2000 g for 3 minutes. (See "Centrifuge Calibration" in this section for more information regarding centrifuge speed and time.)

💣 Once centrifugation has ceased, it is important to allow the centrifuge to stop spinning without operator intervention, any acute stop of the rotor, including brake use, will disturb the red cell/plasma line thereby contaminating the plasma with red cells.

# Component Separation

7. The unit of whole blood should be removed from the centrifuge without agitation so as not to disturb red cells and plasma and placed on a plasma extractor (Fenwal; Plasma Separation Stand, Terumo®.)

✓ The plasma extractor provides a rigid stand in which to place units of whole blood. A hinged plate is attached to the stand and may be released to apply pressure to the unit of whole blood in order to express the plasma into a satellite bag (see Figure 2-8).

8. One empty satellite bag should be placed on a balance. The weight should be tared to zero. The Platelet Rich Plasma will be expressed into the empty satellite bag.

♥ The number of integrally attached satellite bags is dependent on the blood collection system being used. For this discussion, a triple bag is used: there are two satellite bags, one contains Adsol®, one is empty.

9. Open the plastic port at the top of the blood collection bag. Remove plasma by releasing the hinged plate of the plasma extractor and applying pressure to the bag containing the centrifuged whole blood. Platelet Rich Plasma will be expressed into the empty satellite bag.

💣 The task of extracting platelets from centrifuged whole blood can be challenging, as red cells lie just below the platelet layer (see Figure 2-12). Platelet Rich Plasma should be light yellow in color and should not contain visible red cell contamination.

10. Using hemostats, clamp off the line of the bag containing the harvested plasma and seal. Process the Red Cells as described on page 77.

## Determine Volume

11. Calculate the volume of Platelet Rich Plasma. Tare the weight of the balance to zero and weigh the Platelet Rich Plasma. The weight of the empty bag should be subtracted from the final weight of the bag. By dividing the final weight of the product by the appropriate specific gravity, the volume in milliliters can be calculated.

✓ The specific gravity of plasma is 1.023, so 1 gram of plasma is approximately equal to 1 milliliter of plasma.

12. The final product should be labeled with the product name and volume in milliliters.

## Storage

13. In order to preserve platelet viability, Platelet Rich Plasma should be allowed to rest at room temperature, label side down, for 1-2 hours and transfused as soon as possible thereafter.

# Crossmatch Procedure

## Principle

✓ The major and minor crossmatch are performed to assist in providing compatible red cell products and possibly alleviating adverse reactions to transfusion.

✓ The major crossmatch is performed to detect antibodies in the recipient's serum that may agglutinate or lyse the donor's erythrocytes.

✓ Conversely, the minor crossmatch detects antibodies in the donor plasma directed against recipient erythrocytes.

✓ The auto control may detect autoantibodies.

# Equipment

Normal Saline

12 x 75 mm test tubes

Centrifuge (Figure 5-1)

Microscope

Agglutination Viewer (Figure 5-2) or well lit area

37° C Heat Block  (Figure 5-3)

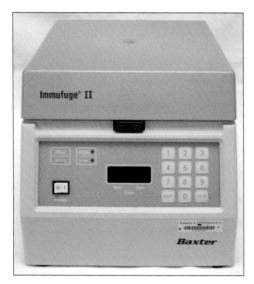

**Figure 5-1** Immufuge.

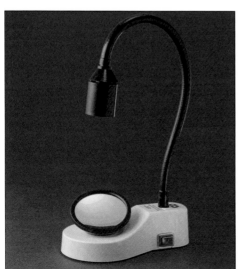

**Figure 5-2** Agglutination viewer. (Image supplied by and used with permission of Fisher Scientific.)

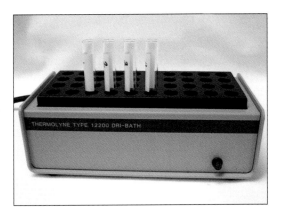

**Figure 5-3** 37° C heat block.

# Procedure

1. Prepare donor and recipient blood samples.

    Donor red cells and plasma or serum:

    For stored whole blood or red cells:

    Donor samples may be obtained by using a segment from the blood bag. This segment is separated from the bag and clipped open. After allowing this sample to drain into a labeled 12 x 75 mm test tube, the donor blood sample should be centrifuged and the supernatant plasma should be separated from the red cells (Figure 5-4).

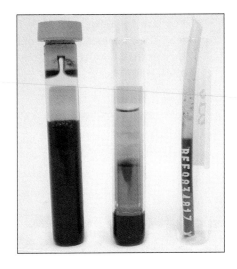

**Figure 5-4** Sources of donor red blood cells.

For blood samples obtained directly from the blood donor:

One 5 ml red top Vacutainer™ tube and one 5 ml EDTA tube are sufficient for compatibility testing. The red top is centrifuged and the serum separated from the red blood cells. The red blood cells may be extracted from the clotted portion of the red top tube or from the EDTA sample.

Recipient red cells and serum:

The blood sample is obtained directly from the recipient:

One 5 ml red top Vacutainer™ tube and one 5 ml EDTA tube are sufficient for compatibility testing. The red top is centrifuged and the serum separated from the red blood cells. The red blood cells may be extracted from the clotted portion of the red top tube or from the EDTA sample.

2. Prepare 3-5% donor and recipient cell suspensions. (See "Washed Cell Suspension", page 87.)

3. Major Crossmatch:

For each donor, label a 12 x 75 mm test tube with the donor number and "major." Add two drops of the patient serum and one drop of the appropriate donor cell suspension.

4. Minor Crossmatch:

For each donor, label a test tube with the donor number and "minor". Add two drops of the appropriate donor serum and one drop of the patient cell suspension.

5. Auto Control:

For the patient and each donor, label a test tube with "AC" and the patient name or donor number. Add two drops of serum and one drop of the corresponding cell suspension for each sample.

In Summary:

| TEST | SERUM/PLASMA | CELLS |
|------|--------------|-------|
| Major Crossmatch | Patient | Donor |
| Minor Crossmatch | Donor | Patient |
| Patient Autocontrol | Patient | Patient |
| Donor Autocontrol | Donor | Donor |

6. Mix all tubes and incubate at 37° C (or species specific "normal" body temperature) for a minimum of 15 minutes.

7. Centrifuge for a saline spin. (See Centrifuge Calibration, page 95.)

8. Read macroscopically. Grade reactions using "Reaction Grading" guidelines (page 88.) Confirm all negative reactions microscopically.

9. Record results.

## Interpretation

♠※ Negative reactions in the major and minor crossmatch indicate compatibility.

♠※ A positive reaction indicates incompatibility.

♠※ Positive auto controls should be investigated. Donors who test auto control positive should be excluded from use.

# Washed Cell Suspension

## Principle

Red blood cell samples used for compatibility testing should be washed free of potentially contaminating substances which may interfere with the testing procedure.

## Reagents

Normal Saline

## Equipment

12 x 75 mm test tubes

Plastic transfer pipettes

Centrifuge

## Procedure

1. Label a 12 x 75-mm tube with appropriate identification.

2. With a pipette, place approximately 250 microliters of red blood cells in the labeled tube.

The red blood cells may be obtained from:

An EDTA blood sample collected from the blood donor

The clotted portion of a red top Vacutainer™ tube collected from the donor, or

A blood bag segment.

3. Fill the tube with approximately 4 mls of normal saline and mix well, preparing a homogeneous suspension of the cells in saline.

4. Centrifuge for a wash spin.

5. Decant or aspirate the supernatant saline from the cells.

6. Repeat steps 3-5 one to three times. The goal is to achieve a clear and colorless supernatant. (Figure 5-5)

7. Reconstitute the washed cells with approximately 3 mls normal saline. This will approximate a 3-5% cell suspension.

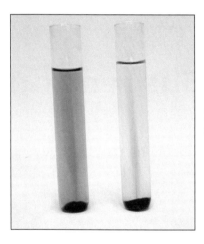

**Figure 5-5** Saline wash supernatant should be colorless and clear (on right).

# Reaction Grading

## Principle

The degree of red cell agglutination and/or hemolysis observed in any blood bank test procedure is significant. The following procedure outlines a system for grading observed test reactions.

## Materials

Centrifuged test specimens to be evaluated

Agglutination viewer or well lit area

# Procedure

1. Remove sample from centrifuge head gently. Do not disturb the cell button.

2. Evaluate the sample for hemolysis by observing the supernatant for the presence of free hemoglobin.

3. Holding the tube under the agglutination viewer (or in well-lit area with a white background), gently shake the tube to disrupt the red blood cell button. This movement should gently move the supernatant back and forth over the cell button using a shaking or tilting motion.

4. Observe the way the red blood cells leave the red cell button.

5. Record the reactivity:

| | |
|---|---|
| 4+ | One solid aggregate of cells |
| 3+ | Several large aggregates |
| 2+ | Large agglutinates and smaller clumps |
| 1+ | Many small agglutinates and a background of free red blood cells |
| +/- Macro | Weak agglutinates seen macroscopically. Many agglutinates microscopically |
| +/- Micro | No agglutinates seen macroscopically. Few agglutinates microscopically |
| H | Hemolysis |
| 0 | Negative. No agglutination observed macroscopically or microscopically. |

Please consult Figure 5-6.

# Interpretation

Any agglutination and/or hemolysis observed indicates a positive reaction. The presence of rouleaux should be confirmed using the "Saline Replacement Procedure" on page 91.

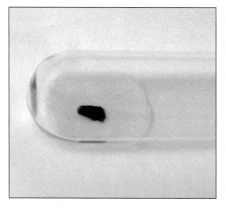

4+ Reaction

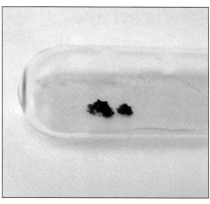

3+ Reaction

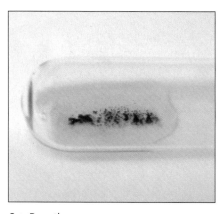

2+ Reaction

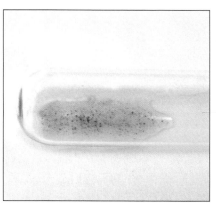

1+ Reaction

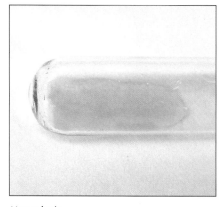

Hemolysis

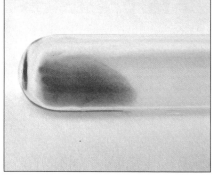

Negative reaction

**Figure 5-6** Reaction grading guidelines.

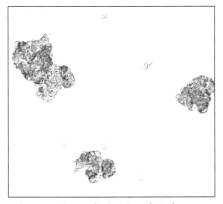

Microscopic agglutination (20X)

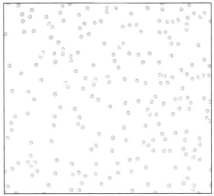

Microscopic negative (20X)

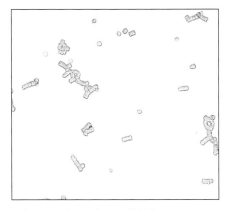

Microscopic rouleaux (20X)

**Figure 5-6** Reaction grading guidelines. (continued)

# Saline Replacement Procedure

## Principle

Red blood cells exhibiting rouleaux appear as "stacked coins" when observed microscopically. Rouleaux formations disperse with the addition of normal saline while true agglutination remains. For compatibility testing, rouleaux is considered a negative reaction. The following procedure is used to distinguish rouleaux from true agglutination.

# Materials

Normal saline

Microscope

Pipette

Microscope slide

# Procedure

1. If rouleaux is suspected, recentrifuge the sample using the saline spin. Decant the serum/plasma (Figure 5-7).

2. To the cell button, add 2 drops of saline. Mix by gentle shaking until the cell button is dispersed.

3. Recentrifuge the sample using the saline spin.

4. Shake the tube and disrupt the red cell button in the tube. Grade reaction accordingly. If no agglutination is observed macroscopically, read microscopically.

5. Record results.

# Interpretation

💣 True rouleaux will disperse with the addition of saline and is NOT considered agglutination.

✓ Rouleaux is commonly exhibited in cats and patients with hyperproteiemia.

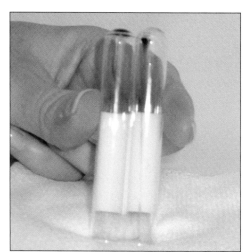

**Figure 5-7** Decanting serum/plasma for saline replacement procedure.

# Warming Whole Blood, Red Cells, or Thawing FFP, Cryo, or Cryo-Poor Plasma

✓ Rapid infusion of cold blood products may cause adverse reactions in the recipient. Therefore, Whole Blood and Red Cells should be warmed prior to transfusion and frozen products must be thawed and warmed before transfusion.

✓ Dry heat devices, countercurrent heat exchange units or circulating water baths may be used to warm blood products.

💣 These devices should not increase the temperature of the red cells to a temperature that causes hemolysis or increases the temperature of plasma products to a temperature that inactivates the viable plasma proteins.

✓ A visible thermometer is useful in monitoring the temperature of the device or an audible alarm that sounds if the specified warming temperature is exceeded.

✓ There are commercially available microwave ovens **specifically designed** for thawing plasma. These devices are **not** designed for use with Red Cells.

✓ A water bath is commonly used for blood warming and plasma thawing. It is important to use a circulating water bath so that water temperature is evenly distributed throughout the bath.

✓ The water temperature should not exceed 37° C (or species specific "normal" body temperature.)

✓ It may be beneficial to set the water bath temperature to a few degrees cooler than the optimal temperature to compensate for any temperature fluctuation that may occur.

✓ The water bath should be clean and free from bacterial contamination.

✓ The blood product should be placed in a zippered closure plastic bag in order to keep the ports of the blood bag free from any possible bacterial contamination from the water bath.

✓ If plastic bags are not used, the ports of the blood bag should be kept above the water line of the water bath to prevent possible contamination. This can be accomplished by using a clean knitting needle or grill skewer threaded through the openings in the top sealed edge of the blood bag (Figure 5-8).

✓ Make sure that blood product is physically separated from the mechanical circulator so that the blood product will not become entangled with and potentially damaged by the circulator.

✓ Do **not** place any blood product at room temperature to warm or thaw.

💣 Remember that blood products are a rich environment for bacterial growth. The process of warming or thawing and subsequent transfusion should occur as quickly as possible.

✓ Red Cells should be transfused immediately after warming for 15-20 minutes. Plasma of volumes of 100-250 mls will thaw within 30-45 minutes and should also be transfused immediately after thawing. Cryo should not be exposed to temperatures of 30-37° C for more than 15 minutes (this minimizes degradation of Factor VIII) and should be transfused immediately after thawing.

✓ A visual check of all blood products should be performed before the unit is transfused. For Red Cell products, clotting, color change to dark purple or black or hemolysis is indicative of bacterial contamination.

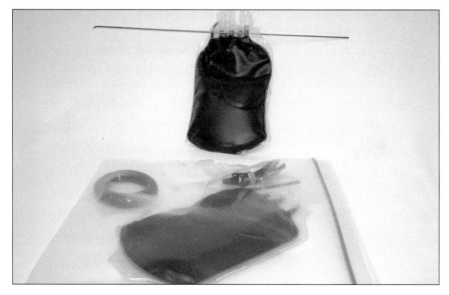

**Figure 5-8** Warming a unit of blood: Ports should be kept free from bacterial contamination. This is best achieved by zippered closure plastic bags or keeping the ports above the water line.

# Centrifuge Calibration

In Blood Banking, centrifuges are used for component preparation and compatibility testing; centrifuge speed and spin times are two important considerations when performing these procedures.

✓ Centrifuge speed is usually specified in component preparation procedures using the value known as relative centrifugal force or rcf.

✓ Centrifuge speed varies by model and manufacturer.

✓ The Immunofuge® is a centrifuge widely used for compatibility testing; centrifuge times in compatibility testing are generally specified for use of this piece of equipment.

✓ Before put in use, centrifuges used for component preparation or compatibility testing should be evaluated to assure quality.

✓ The following procedure will outline the process of centrifuge calibration for component preparation and serologic testing. Once the spin times are established, they should be confirmed annually and after centrifuge repair or adjustment.

## Centrifuge Calibration for Component Preparation

✓ Blood components are prepared by separation of whole blood; this process can be accelerated by the use of a centrifuge.

✓ Centrifuge time and speed are dependent on what types of blood components are to be made.

- A 5-minute heavy spin (5000g) is required for preparation of Red Cells.

- A three minute light spin (2000g) is used in preparation of Platelet Rich Plasma.

♥ Centrifuge times that are given include acceleration time, but do not include deceleration time.

✓ Relative centrifugal force (in g) is calculated using the following formula:

RCF (in g) = 28.38 X radius of centrifuge rotor in inches X $(rpm/1000)^2$

✓ Evaluation of the heavy spin time is achieved by performing quality control on the components that are made.

✓ Red Cells should be evaluated by confirming the final hematocrit of the unit.

✓ Cryoprecipitate should be evaluated by confirming fibrinogen and Factor VIII activity.

✓ Spin times may be increased or decreased according to the outcome of these tests.

✓ Revolutions per minute (rpm) may be confirmed using a Tachometer.

# Centrifuge Calibration for Compatibility Testing

✓ Calibration of centrifuges used for serologic testing is performed in order to assure that spin times do not cause either false positive or false negative results. The following procedures should be used to confirm calibration in a new centrifuge, annually or after any adjustment or repair.

💣 **Please note that red cell behavior is evaluated, NOT reaction strength.**

## Saline Spin

In compatibility testing, red cells that are suspended in saline require a centrifuge time based on red cell reactivity in this medium. The following procedure establishes the saline spin time.

### Materials Needed

Serum that will produce a 1+ reaction

Two 3 - 5% red cell samples:

"Positive" – Red cells that will react with the above serum sample

"Negative" – Red cells that will not react with the above serum sample

12 x 75 mm test tubes

Pipettes

Agglutination viewer or well lit area

Centrifuge

### Procedure

1. Place ten 12 x 75 mm test tubes in a rack. Place two drops of serum in each tube.

2. In 5 of these tubes, add one drop of the "Negative" red cells.

3. In the other 5 tubes, add one drop of the "Positive" red cells.

4. There are now 5 pairs of tubes, each containing one negative and one positive sample.

Centrifuge one pair for 10 seconds, one pair for 15 seconds, one pair for 20 seconds, one pair for 30 seconds and one pair for 40 seconds. Record results on a worksheet similar to the one shown in Table 5-1.

### Table 5-1  Serologic Centrifuge Calibration Worksheet

For Saline Spin Time:

| TIME IN SECONDS | SUPERNATANT CLEAR? | CELL BUTTON CLEARLY DELINEATED? | CELLS EASILY RESUSPENDED? | POSITIVE IS POSITIVE? | NEGATIVE IS NEGATIVE? |
|---|---|---|---|---|---|
| 10 | | | | | |
| 15 | | | | | |
| 20 | | | | | |
| 30 | | | | | |
| 40 | | | | | |

For Wash Spin Time:

| TIME IN SECONDS | SUPERNATANT CLEAR? | CELL BUTTON CLEARLY DELINEATED? |
|---|---|---|
| 30 | | |
| 45 | | |
| 60 | | |
| 90 | | |
| 120 | | |

## Interpretation

The centrifuge time that should be used for a Saline Spin is the shortest centrifuge time that fulfills the following criteria (as specified by the American Association of Blood Banks):

1. The positive tube is 1+ positive.

2. The negative tube is negative.

3. The cell button is clearly delineated.

4. The supernatant is clear.

5. The cell button can be easily resuspended.

**NOTE:** If additives (such as albumin or low ionic strength saline) are used in crossmatching, this procedure may be modified to establish spin times. This should be done in a procedure separate from establishing the Saline Spin. A set of five paired samples should be set up as outlined in the procedure above.  The appropriate additive should be incubated with each pair for the appropriate incubation time and then evaluated for spin time.

# Wash Spin

Red cells used for compatibility testing should be washed in order to remove potentially contaminating substances, which may interfere with the testing procedure.  The following procedure establishes the centrifuge time for the Wash Spin.

## Materials Needed

EDTA Blood specimen with a normal hematocrit

Normal saline

12 x 75 mm test tubes

Pipettes

Agglutination viewer or well lit area

Centrifuge

## Procedure

1.  Place five 12 x 75 mm test tubes in a rack.

2.  Add at least 250 microliters of the EDTA blood specimen to each tube.

3.  Add approximately 4 mls of normal saline to each tube. Mix well for homogeneity.

4.  Centrifuge one tube for 30 seconds (remember to balance!), one tube for 45 seconds, one tube for 60 seconds, one tube for 90 seconds and one tube for 120 seconds. Record results on a worksheet similar to Table 5-1.

## Interpretation

The centrifuge time that should be used as the Wash Spin is the shortest centrifuge time that fulfills the following criteria:

1.  The supernatant is clear.

2.  The cell button is clearly delineated.

3.  The red cells are in a compact button.

## Results

Spin times should be posted and/or included in procedures to ensure consistency in testing.

# Appendix 1: Manufacturers of Blood Collection Bags

**For Dogs:**

Baxter Fenwal
1627 Lake Cook Road
Deerfield, IL 60015
Telephone: (800) 766-1077
http://www.baxterfenwal.com

Terumo Medical Corporation
2101 Cottontail Lane
Somerset, NJ 08873
Telephone: (800) 283-7866
http://www.terumomedical.com

Haemonetics Corporation
400 Wood Road
Braintree, MA 02184-9114
Telephone: (781) 848-7100
http://www.haemonetics.com

**For Cats:**

Animal Blood Bank
P.O.Box 118
Dixon, CA 65620
Telephone: (800) 243-5759
http://www.animalbloodbank.com

# Appendix 2: Organizations with Veterinary Blood Bank Interests

Animal Blood Bank
P.O.Box 118
Dixon, CA 65620
Telephone: (800) 243-5759
http://www.animalbloodbank.com

Eastern Veterinary Blood Bank
808 Bestgate Road
Suite 111
Annapolis, MD 21401
Telephone: 800-949-EVBB
http://www.evbb.com

Hemopet Blood Bank
11330 Markon Drive
Garden Grove, CA 92841 USA
Phone: 714-891-2022
http://www.hemopet.com

# Index

## A

ABO compatibility, 46

Additives, 17
  in blood collection systems, 20

Adsol (AS-1), 17, 20
  in component separation, 77-78
  in separation of platelet rich plasma components, 82

Agglutination viewer, 84, 89

Albumin, 48
  for hypooncotic patients, 49
  in plasma, 24

Allergic reactions, 55, 57-58

Alloimmunization, 60

Aluminum sealing clip, 11

Antibody formation, 60

Antibody screening cells, 46-47

Anticoagulant-citrate-dextrose (ACD), 19

Anticoagulant-preservatives, 16-17
  in blood product preparation, 75
  in canine blood collection systems, 19-20
  decreasing amount of, 39-40
  removal of, 40

Anticoagulants, 16-17
  in feline blood collection systems, 20
  in open canine blood collection systems, 18-19

Auto control, 86

Autoantibodies, detecting, 83

## B

Balancing devices, 30

Biochemical profile, 6-7

Biohazards, disposal of, 65

Biosafety, 64-71

Blood administration sets, 54-55

Blood bags
  centrifugation of, 31
  identification numbers for, 27
  removing anticoagulant-preservative from, 40
  sealing of, 27, 28
  short draw, 23

Blood bank organizations, 100

Blood banks
  indelible records for, 68
  quality indicators for, 66-67
  records related to, 68-69

Blood cells, sensitization to, 48

Blood collection
  equipment for, 10-12
  short draw, 39

Blood collection bags, 10-11
  manufacturers of, 99

Blood collection systems, 26-27
  canine, 18-20
  closed, 19-21
  feline, 20-21
  open, 18-19, 20
  pre-processing guidelines for, 27-28

Blood components
  physiologic functions of, 49
  quality control of, 67
  separation of, 31-33

Blood donor programs
  incentives for, 4
  recruiting owners into, 4-5

Blood donors
  blood samples from, 86
  keeping track of, 10
  laboratory evaluation of, 7-9
  physical attributes of, 5-6
  scheduling for phlebotomy, 10
  selection of, 9

Blood draw volume, optimum, 27

Blood products, 21-26. *See also* specific products
   additives in, 17
   anticoagulant-preservatives for, 16-17
   determining volume of, 78
   feline, 78
   guidelines for issuing, 71
   increasing oxygen transport, 50
   inventory management of, 69-71
   limited resources of, 48
   optimal stock levels of, 70
   ordering guidelines for, 70
   packaging of, 43
   preparation of, 74-78
   preparing for shipment, 42-43
   purchasing, 40-41
   receiving, 42
   shelf life of, 18
   storage of, 33-35, 78
   warming of, 93-94
Blood products scale, 13
Blood separation, equipment for, 13
Blood storage, 33-35
   equipment for, 14
Blood substitutes, 51-53
Blood transfusion. *See also* Transfusion reactions
   adverse effects of, 48, 55-61
   decision for, 49
   guidelines for, 47-50
   for increased oxygen transport, 49-50
   IV solutions interfering with, 53
   kinetic considerations in, 48
   rationale for, 47-48
Blood types, crossmatching, 46-47
Blood volume
   determining, 78
   loss of, 48
Blood warming, 93-94

# C

Calcium, chelation of, 19
Canine blood donors
   attributes of, 5-6
   laboratory evaluation of, 7-8
Canine blood groups, 7, 8
Canine phlebotomy, 10
Canine whole blood, preparation of, 29, 74-75
Centrifugation, 31
   of platelet rich plasma, 37-38, 82
   preparation for, 30
   preparing platelet rich plasma for, 81
   preparing red cells and plasma for, 75-76
   of red cells and plasma, 76-77
Centrifuge, 84
   balanced, 30
   calibration of
      for compatibility testing, 96-98
      for component preparation, 95-96
   refrigerated, 13
   speed of, 95
Chemical plan, 64-65
Circulatory overload, 58
Citrate, 16-17
   intoxication from, 59
   in open canine blood collection systems, 19
Citrate-phosphate-dextrose-adenine (CPDA1), 16-17
   in canine blood collection systems, 19
   in feline blood collection systems, 20
Citrate-phosphate-dextrose (CPD), 16-17
Citrate-phosphate-double-dextrose (CP2D), 16-17
   in canine blood collection systems, 19

Clinical considerations, 46-61

Clotting factor deficiencies, 24

Colloid oncotic pressure (COP), maintaining, 49

Colloids, 49
advantages and contraindications of, 53

Communication
in blood donor recruitment, 4
with blood products supplier, 41

Compatibility testing, centrifuge calibration for, 96-98

Component preparation, centrifuge calibration for, 95-96

Component separation
of canine red cells and fresh frozen plasma, 77-78
of platelet rich plasma, 37-38, 82-83

Countercurrent heat exchange units, 93

Crossmatch
equipment for, 84-85
interpreting, 87
principles of, 83
procedure for, 85-87

Crossmatching, 46-47

Cryo-poor plasma, 25
canine, 79-80
contents and storage of, 22
preparation of, 35-36
separation of, 79-80
thawing of, 93-94

Cryoprecipitate, 36
analysis of, 67
canine, 79-80
expiration of, 80
separation of, 79-80
thawing of, 93-94

Cryoprecipitate-poor plasma. *See* Cryo-poor plasma

Cryoprecipitated antihemophilic factor, 25

contents and storage of, 22
preparation of, 35-36

**D**

Delayed hemolytic reaction, 59

Dextrose, 53

Disseminated intravascular coagulation (DIC), 57

Dog Erythrocyte Antigen (DEA), 7, 8

Donor records, 68

Donor red blood cells, sources of, 85

Dry heat devices, 93

**E**

Electric Heat Sealers, 11

Electrolyte disturbances, 58-59

Epinephrine, 58

Equipment
for crossmatching, 84-85
quality control of, 67
for washed cell suspension, 87

Ergonomic workstations, 65

Erythropoietin, 49

Eye Wash Station, 65

**F**

Factor VIII, 67

Febrile reactions, 55, 57

Fees, for blood donation, 5

Feline AB mis-matched transfusions, 56

Feline blood donors
attributes of, 6
laboratory evaluation of, 9

Feline blood groups, 9

Feline phlebotomy, 11

Feline whole blood, preparation of, 29, 75

Freezer, for blood storage, 14

Frequently Asked Questions brochure, 4

Fresh frozen plasma (FFP), 24
  contents and storage of, 22
  cryoprecipitated anti-hemophilic factor and cryo-poor plasma from, 35-36
  preparation of, 29-30, 74-78
  thawing of, 93-94

Fresh whole blood, 22-23
  contents and storage of, 22
  preparation of, 29, 74-75

Frozen plasma
  monitoring storage of, 34
  purchasing, 42
  storage of, 14, 34

# G

Glass bottles, 19
Graft vs. host reaction, 59-60
Gravity Drip, 54

# H

Hand sealer, 11, 12
Hazardous materials, disposal of, 65
Heat block, 85
Heat seal, 27
Hematocrit
  low, 49-50
  post-transfusion, 50
Hematron Seal Rite, 12
Hemoglobin based solutions, 51-52
Hemogram profile, 6-7
Hemolysis, intravascular, 57
Hemolytic reactions, 56-57
Heparin, 19
Hetastarch, 52-53
  advantages and contraindications of, 53
Homeostatic mechanisms, 48
Hypocalcemia, 59

Hypooncotic patients, 49
Hypothermia, 58

# I

Immunoglobulins, 24
Immunosuppressive therapy, 60
Infection, transmission of, 61
Infectious diseases, 6
Intravascular volume maintenance, 49
Intravenous solutions, compatible, 53
Inventory management, 69-71

# K

Kinetics, blood, 48

# L

Laboratory
  records related to, 69
  safety of, 64-65
Laboratory evaluation, 6-7
  canine, 7-8
  feline, 9
Lactated ringer's solution, 53

# M

Major crossmatch, 46, 86
  negative reactions in, 87
Material Safety Data Sheets (MSDS), 64
  with chemical plan, 65
Minor crossmatch, 86
  negative reactions in, 87
Minor crossmatch test, 46-47

# N

Nutricel (AS-3), 20

# O

Optisol (AS-5), 17, 20
Owner
    attributes of, 5
    recruitment of, 4-5
Oxygen transport, 49
    increasing, 49-50
    products increasing, 50
Oxyglobin Solution, 52

# P

Packaging procedures, 43
Packed cells, 23-24
    contents and storage of, 22
    increasing oxygen transport, 50
Phlebotomy
    equipment for, 10-14
    scheduling donors for, 10
Phlebotomy line, clearing, 27-28
Plasma, 24-25. See also *components of*; Cryo-poor plasma; Fresh frozen plasma (FFP); Frozen plasma
    component separation of, 77-78
    contents and storage of, 22
    harvested, 32
        component separation in, 31-33
    preparation of, 74-75
    shelf life of, 24-25
    storage of, 33-35
    thawing of, 93-94
Plasma expanders, 52
Plasma extractor, 13, 31, 37, 77
    in cryoprecipitate separation, 79
    in separation of platelet rich plasma components, 82
Plasma products, 24-26
Plasma separation, 78
    canine, 78
Plasma substitutes, 52-53
Platelet concentrates, 25-26
Platelet rich plasma, 25

    centrifugation of, 82
        preparation for, 81
    component separation of, 37-38, 82-83
    contents and storage of, 22
    determining volume of, 83
    preparation of, 80-83
        for centrifugation, 37
    separation of, 81-82
    storage of, 38, 83
Polymerized stroma-free hemoglobin, 51-52
Post-transfusion purpura, 60
Pre-processing guidelines, 27-28
Preservatives, 16-17
Product log, 35

# Q

Quality assurance
    definition of, 65-66
    purpose of, 66-67
Quality assurance team, 66
Quality indicators, 66-67

# R

Reaction grading, 88-91
Reagents, 87
Records, 67
    attributes of, 68
    for blood bank, 68-69
    storage of, 69
Red blood cell button, 89
Red blood cell products, 22-24
Red blood cell substitutes, 51-52
Red blood cells, 23-24
    additives to, 23, 24
    canine
        centrifugation of, 76-77
        component separation of, 77-78
        preparation for centrifugation

of, 75-76

contents and storage of, 22

expired, 67

half-inactivation time of, 48

increasing oxygen transport, 50

loss of, 48

preparation of, 29-30, 75-78
  with known packed cell
    volume, 32

recipient, 86

refrigeration of, 16

separation of, 81-82

sources of, 85

storage of, 33-35

warming, 93-94

washed, 87-88

Red cell antigens, sensitization to, 47

Red cell transfusion, 49

Refrigeration
  for blood storage, 33-35
  of red cells, 16

Refrigerator, 14

Rh system, 46

Rouleaux, 89, 91, 92

S

Safety plan, in laboratories, 64-65

Saline replacement procedure, 91-92

Saline spin, 87, 96-98

Saline wash supernatant, 88

Satellite bags, 27
  in blood component separation, 31-32
  in platelet rich plasma separation, 37-38

Scale, for blood products, 13

Serofuge, 84

Serologic centrifuge calibration worksheet, 97

Serum/plasma, decanting, 92

Shelf life, 18

Shipment, 42-43

Short draw, 39

Small animal double syringe collection set, 21

Sodium chloride injection, 53

Sodium citrate, 19

Storage
  of cryoprecipitate and cryo poor plasma, 80
  of platelet rich plasma, 38, 83
  of records, 69
  of red cells and fresh frozen plasma, 78

Suppliers
  communicating with, 41
  identifying, 40-41

Syringe Push, 54-55

T

Temperature monitoring devices, 41

Tissue hypoxia, 49

Transfusion reactions
  allergic, 55, 57-58
  to cold blood product infusion, 93
  delayed immunologic, 59-60
  delayed nonimmunologic, 61
  febrile, 55, 57
  grading, 88-91
  hemolytic, 56-57
  immediate nonimmunologic, 58-59
  signs of, 55-56

Transfusion records, 69

Transfusion service
  indelible records for, 68
  quality assurance in, 66

Transport containers, 43

Tube stripper, 11, 12

# V

Vacutainer tube, 88

Vacuum chamber, 11

VetaPlasma, 53

Veterinary blood bank

    identifying and purchasing from, 40-41

    organizations of, 100

Vitamin K dependent factors, 24

Volume expanders, 52

# W

Wash spin, 98

Washed cell suspension, 87-88

Water bath, 93

Whole blood. *See also* Fresh whole blood

    contents and storage of, 22

    increasing oxygen transport, 50

    preparation of, 29-30

    products of, 22-24

    stored, 23

    warming, 93-94

# Notes

# Notes

# Notes

T - #0728 - 101024 - C120 - 215/146/5 - SB - 9781893441040 - Gloss Lamination